Cancer is a disease that make some of your cells in your body turn bad.

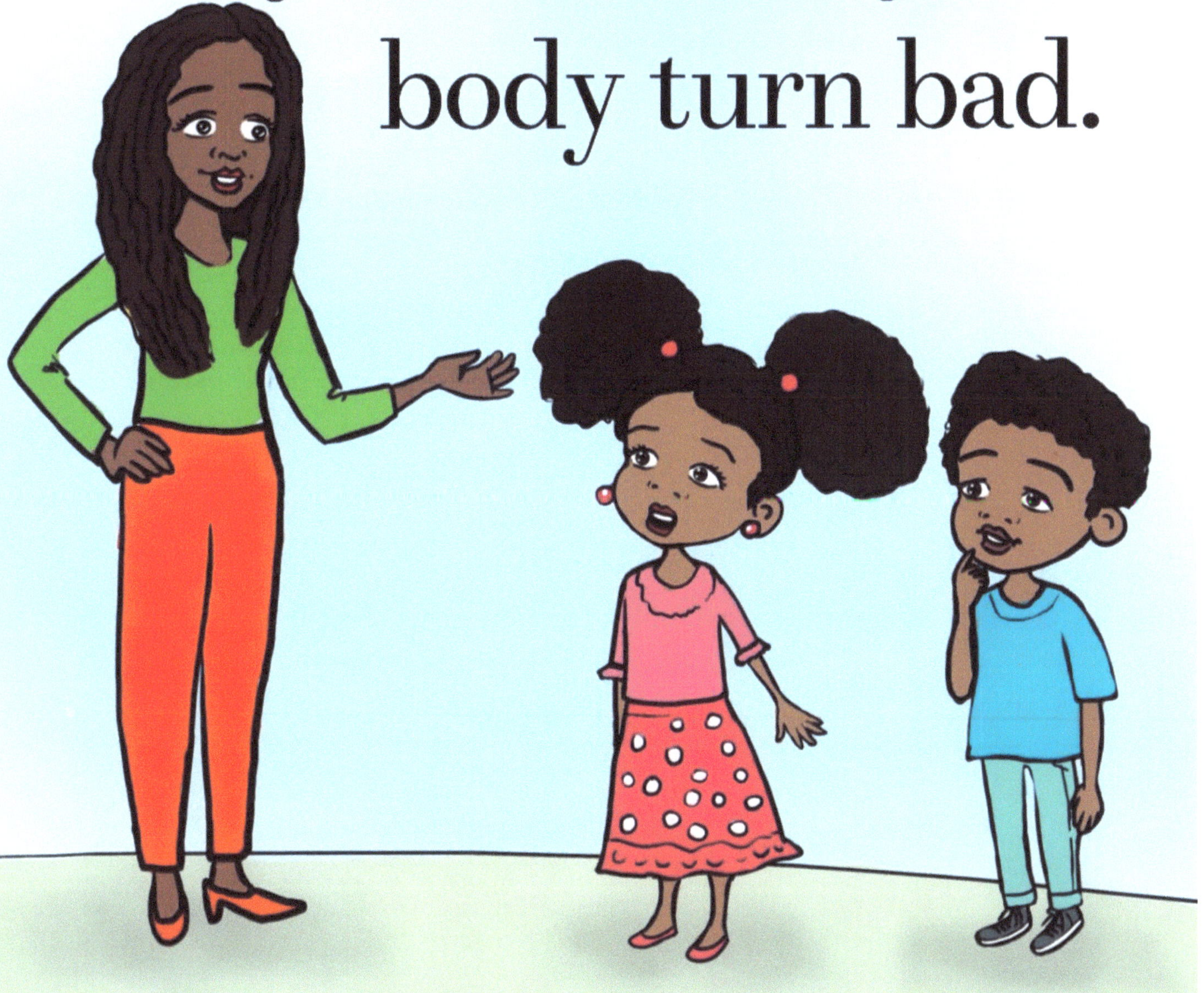

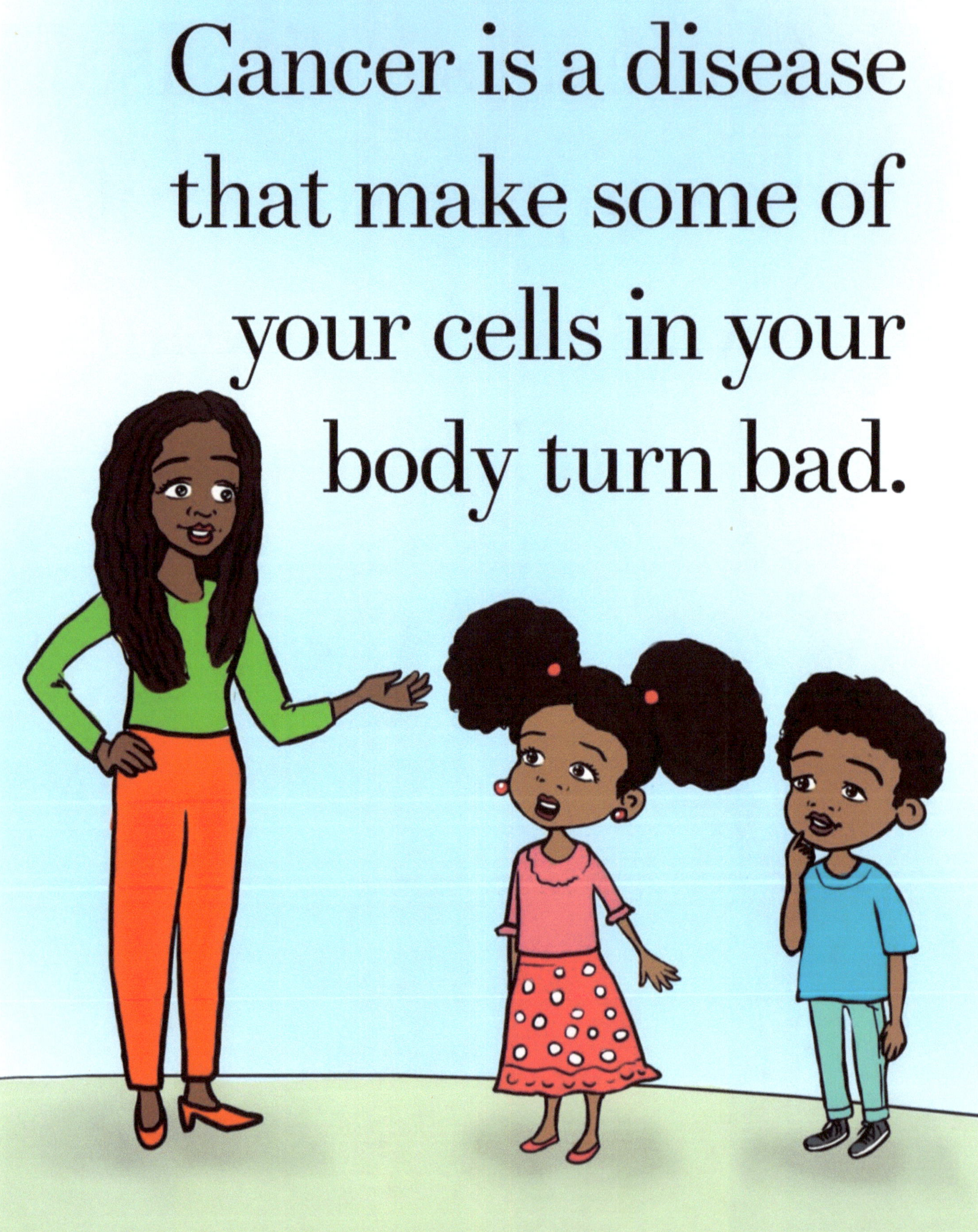
Cancer is a disease that make some of your cells in your body turn bad.

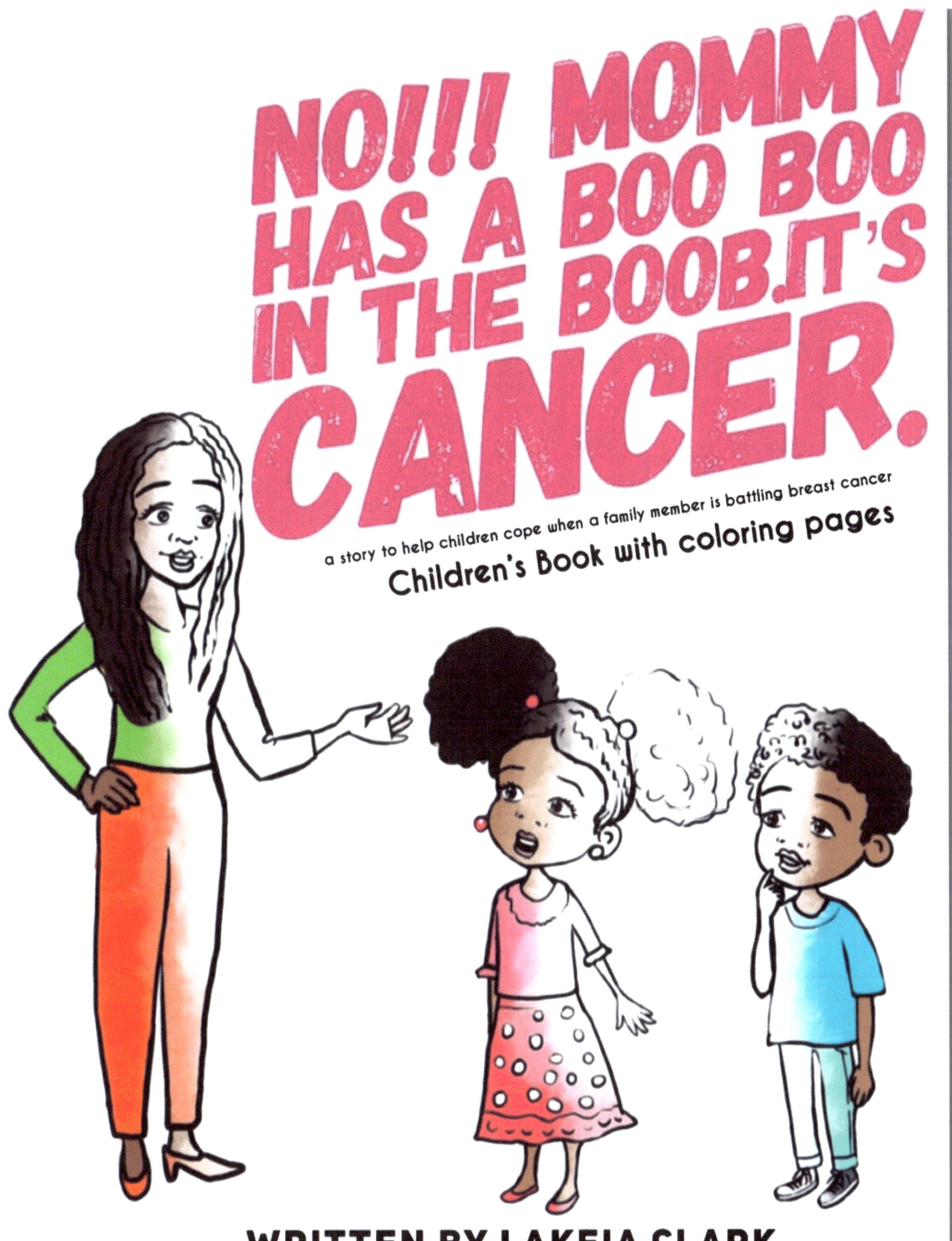

NO!!! MOMMY HAS A BOO BOO IN THE BOOB. IT'S CANCER.
a story to help children cope when a family member is battling breast cancer
Children's Book with coloring pages
WRITTEN BY LAKEIA CLARK
illustrated by Hatice B.

Hey kids, Mommy have something to tell you. I have cancer. I have breast cancer. There is a boo boo in the boob.

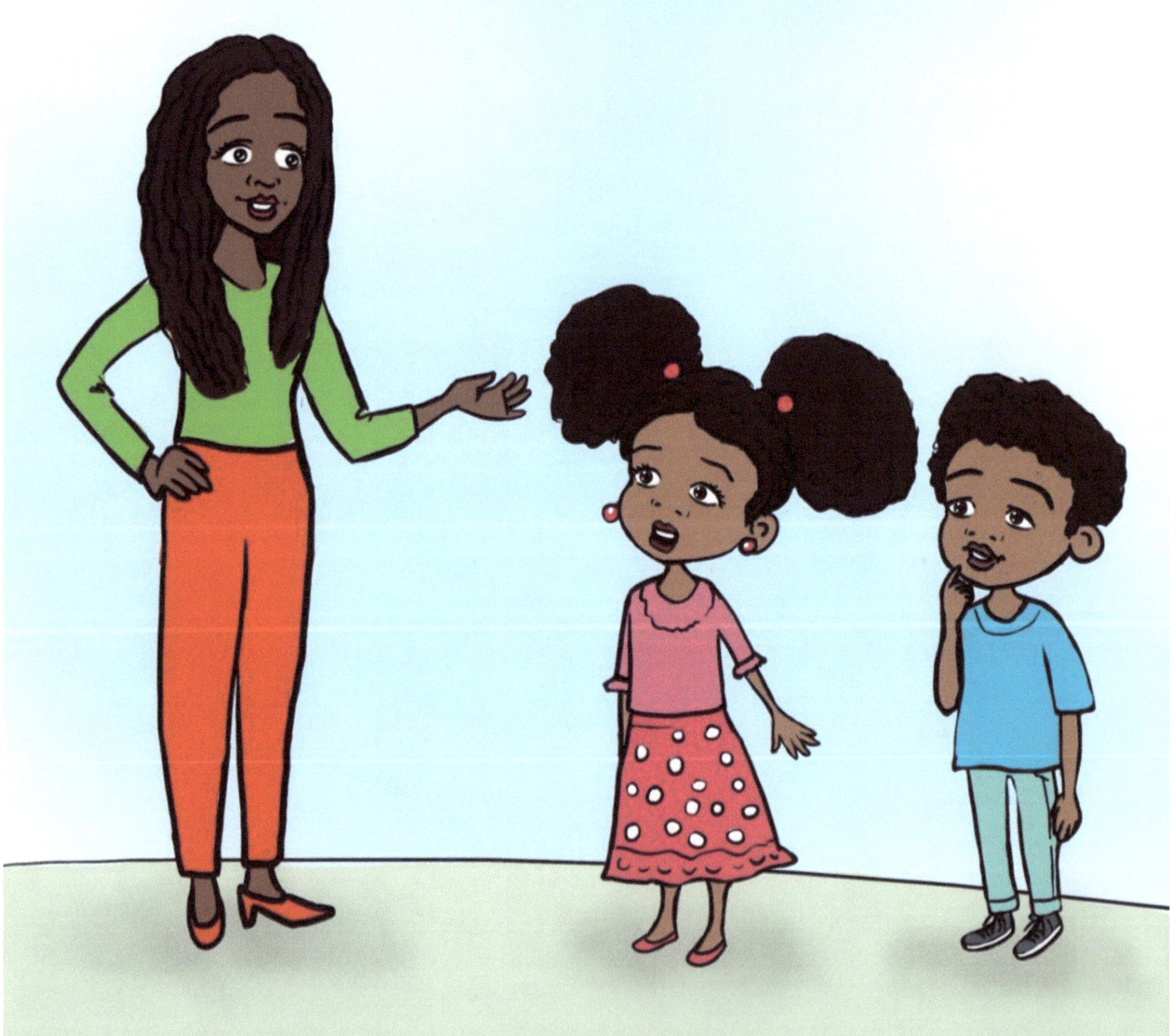

These bad cells grow so
fast that they outgrow
the good cells.Mommy's
bad cells grew into a
lump.The lump is in my boob.

Good Cells And Bad Cells

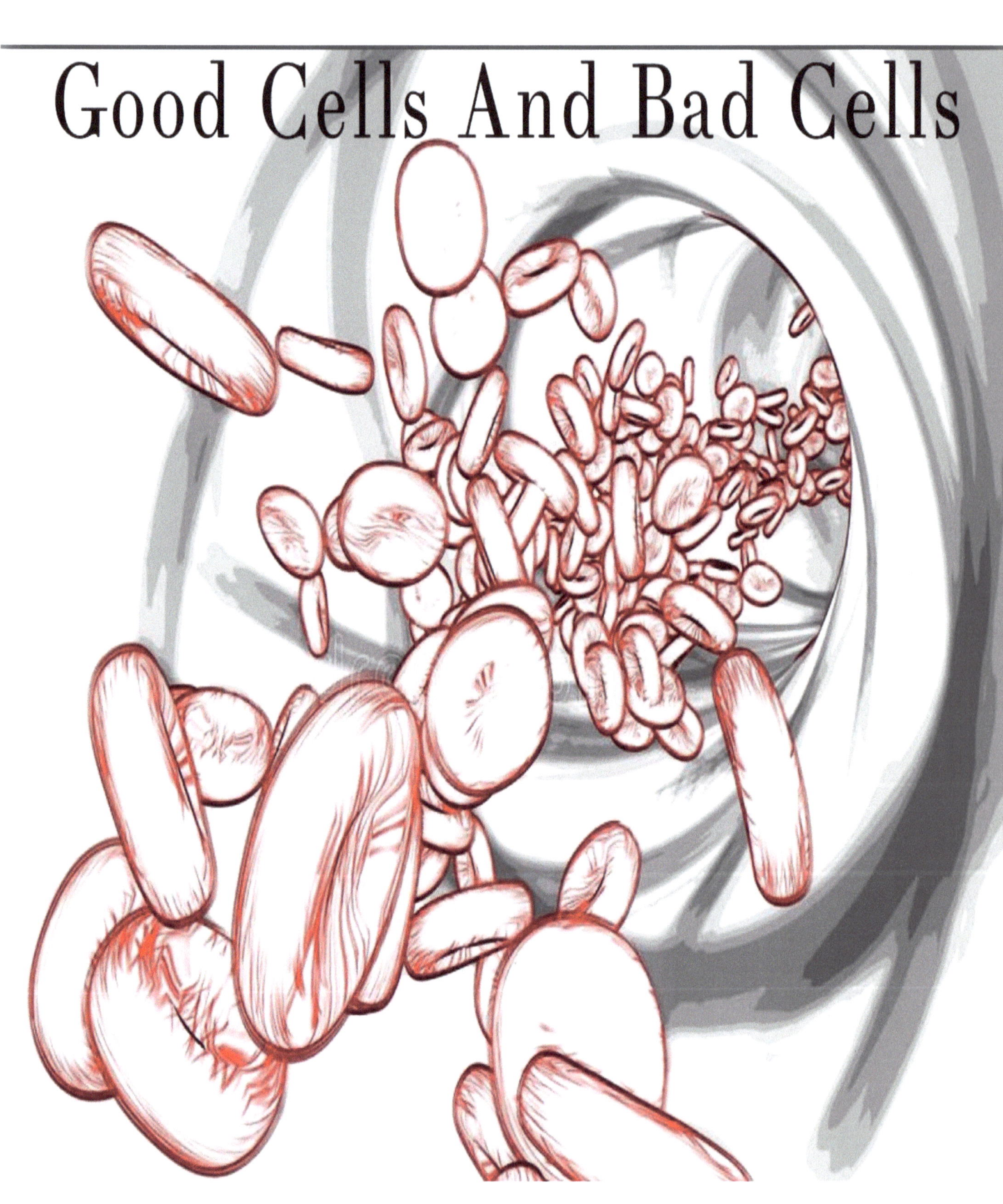

Aww, Mommy do you have a boo boo in the boob?

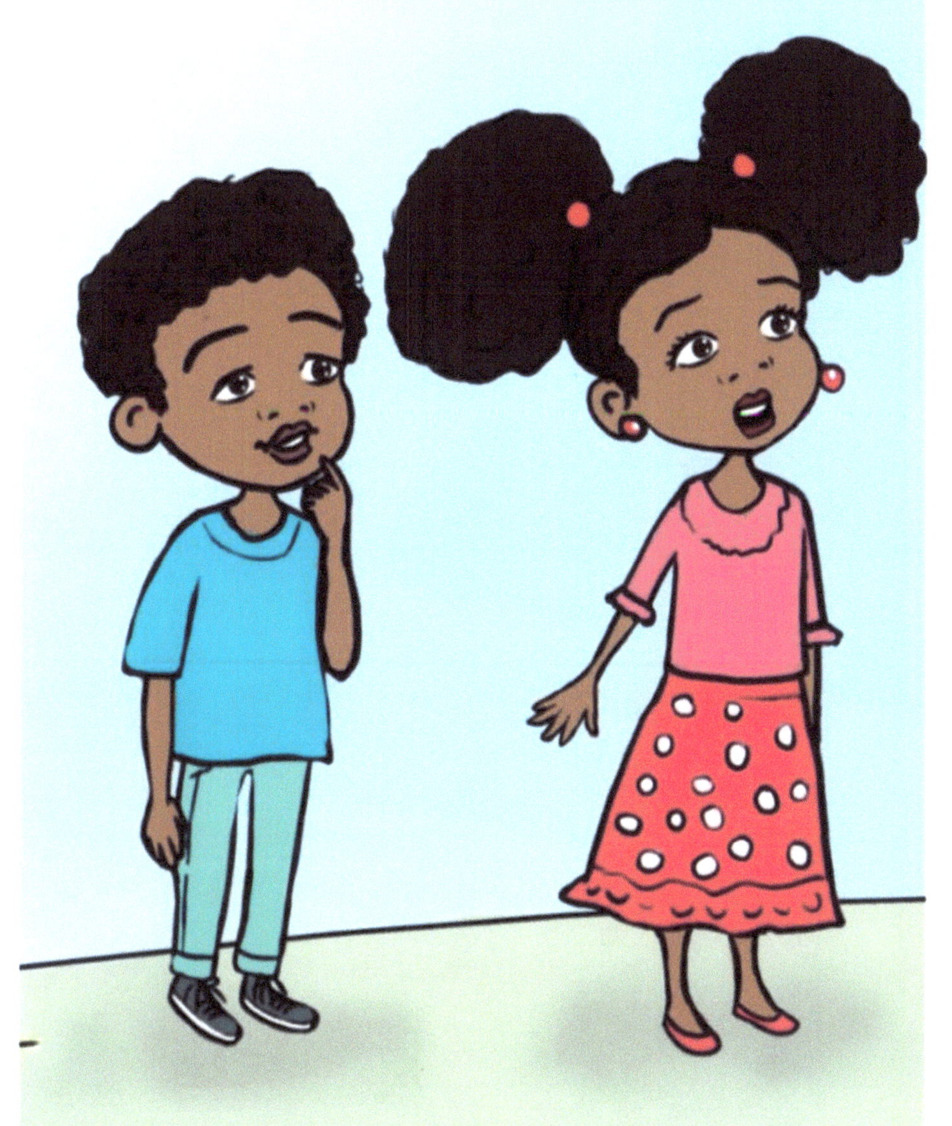

Yes, I do have a boo boo in the boob. However, mommy will be okay.

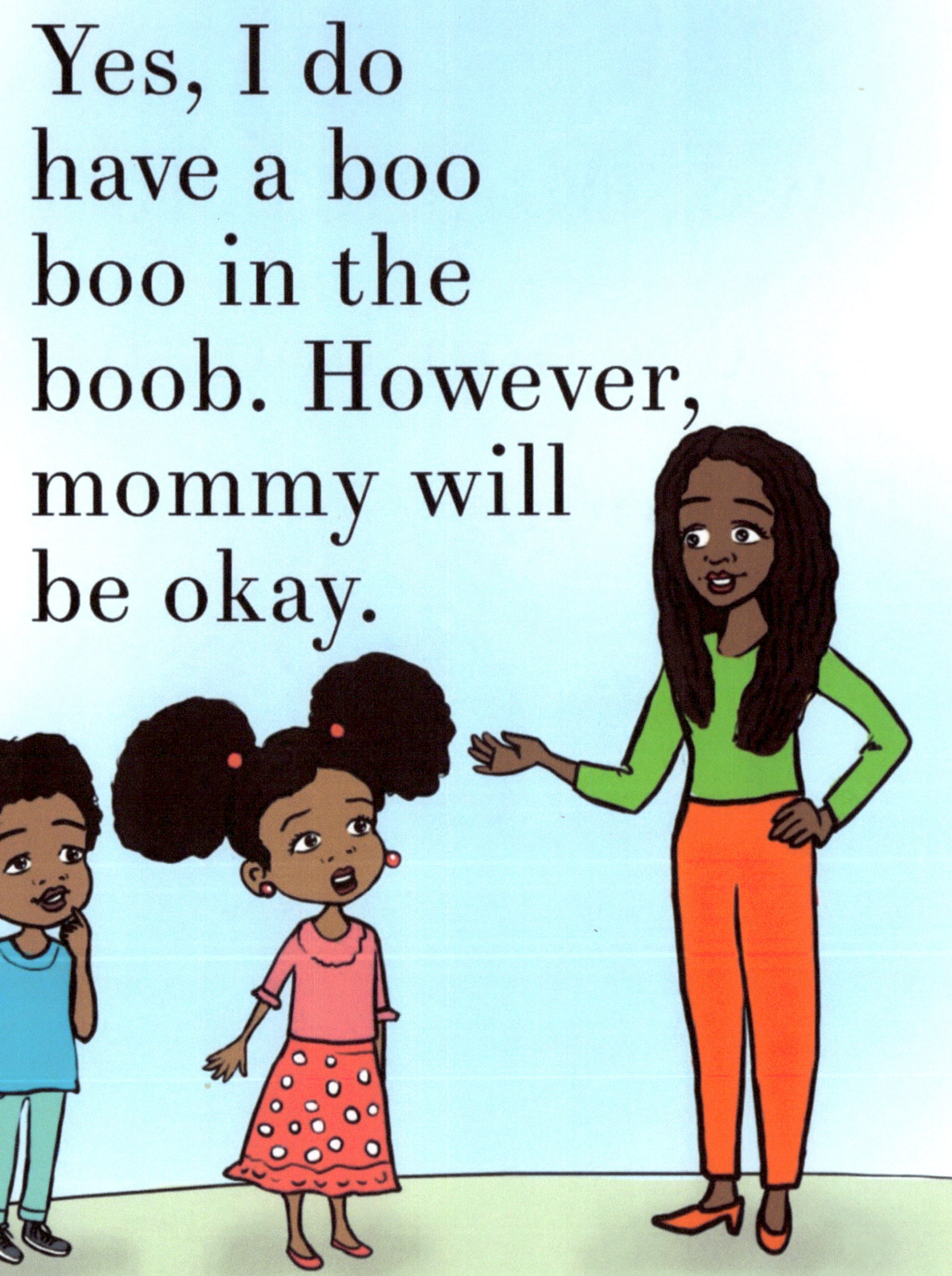

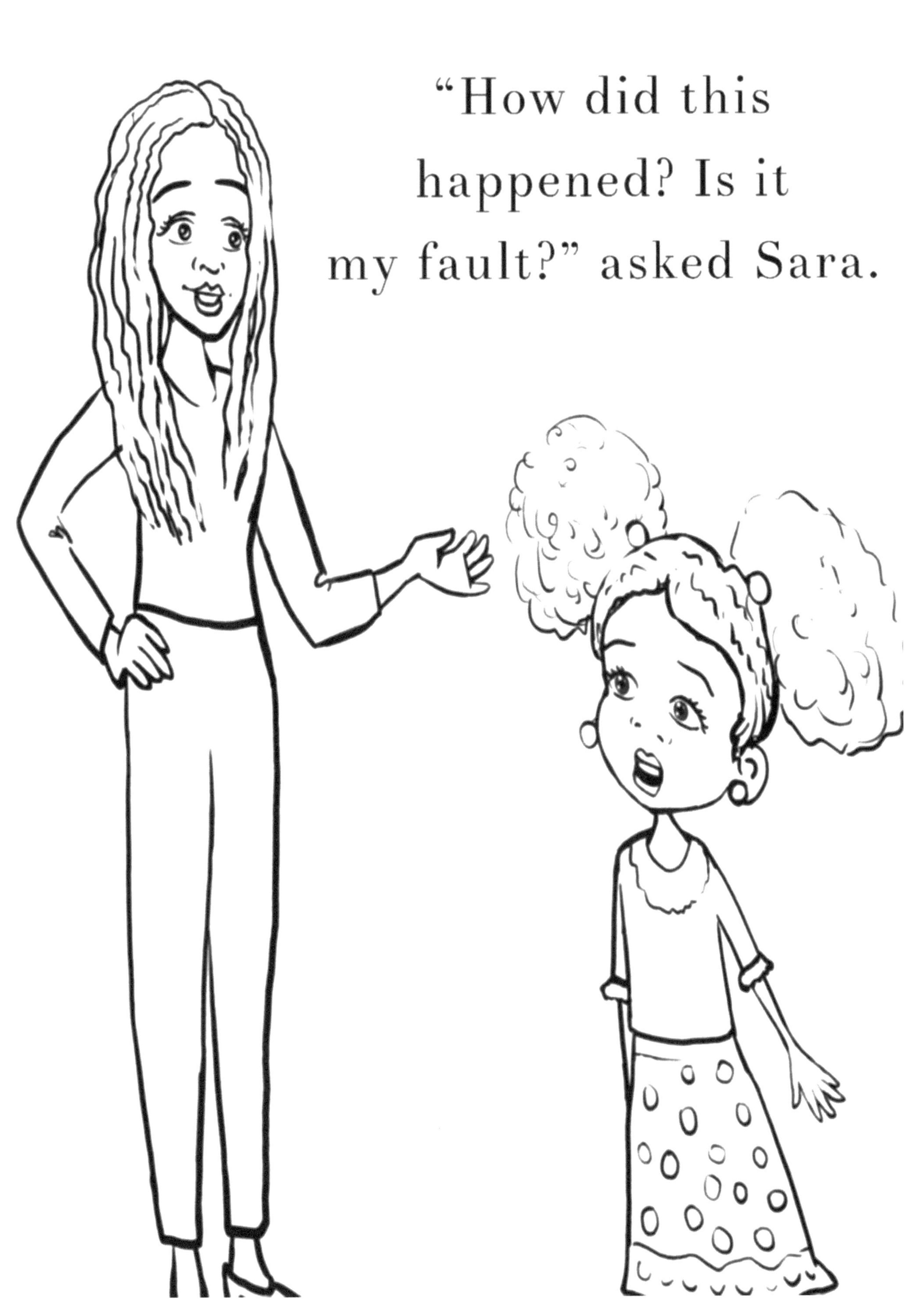

"How did this happened? Is it my fault?" asked Sara.

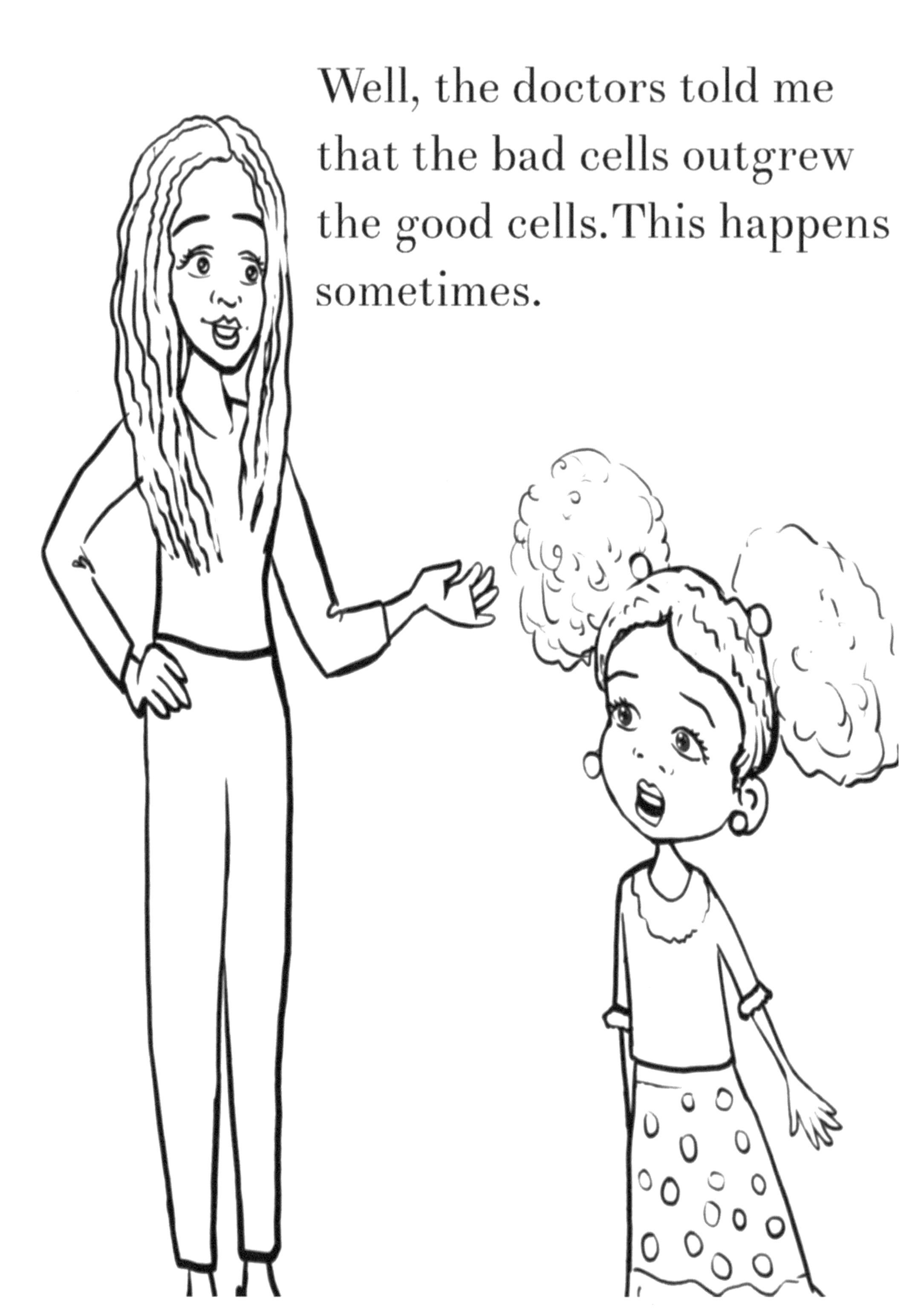

Well, the doctors told me that the bad cells outgrew the good cells. This happens sometimes.

It is not your fault. There is nothing you did to cause the cancer. Cancer does not appear because you did not do your homework. Cancer does not appear because you misbehaved.

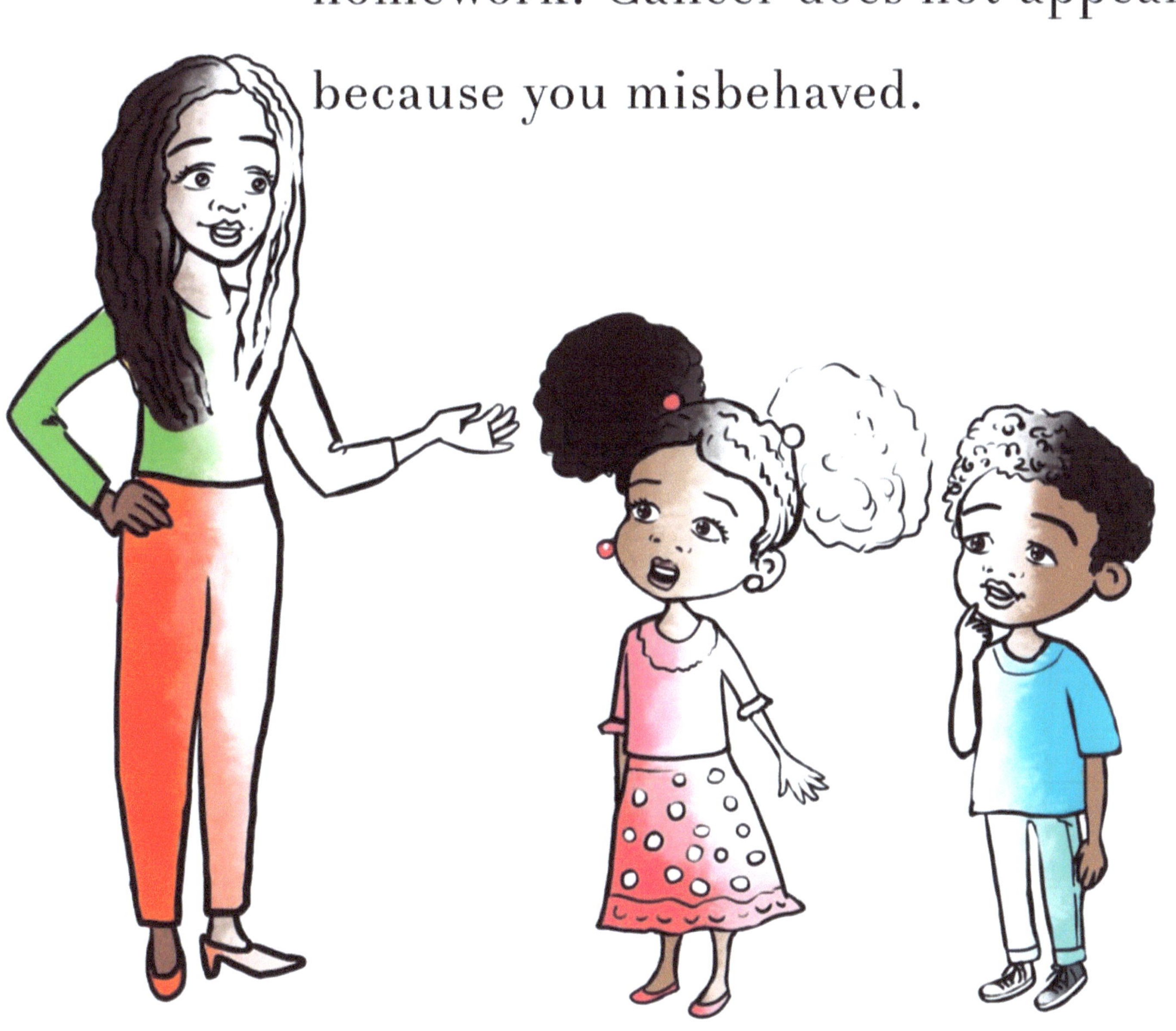

The boo boo in mommy's boob is not my fault either. Sometimes God just entrusts us with hard task in life, and those tasks can encourage someone else to never give up.

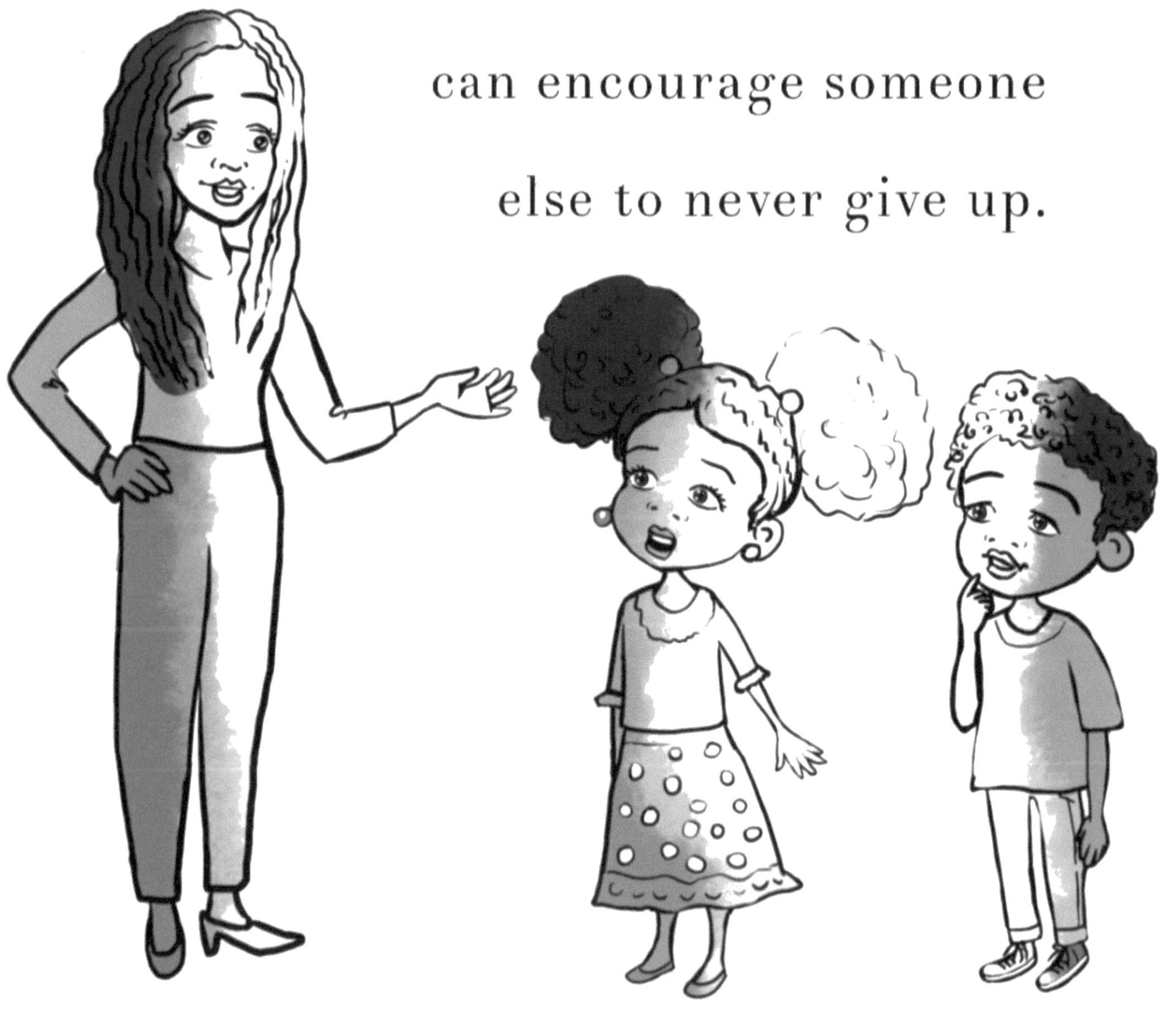

Sara let's allow mommy to get some rest.

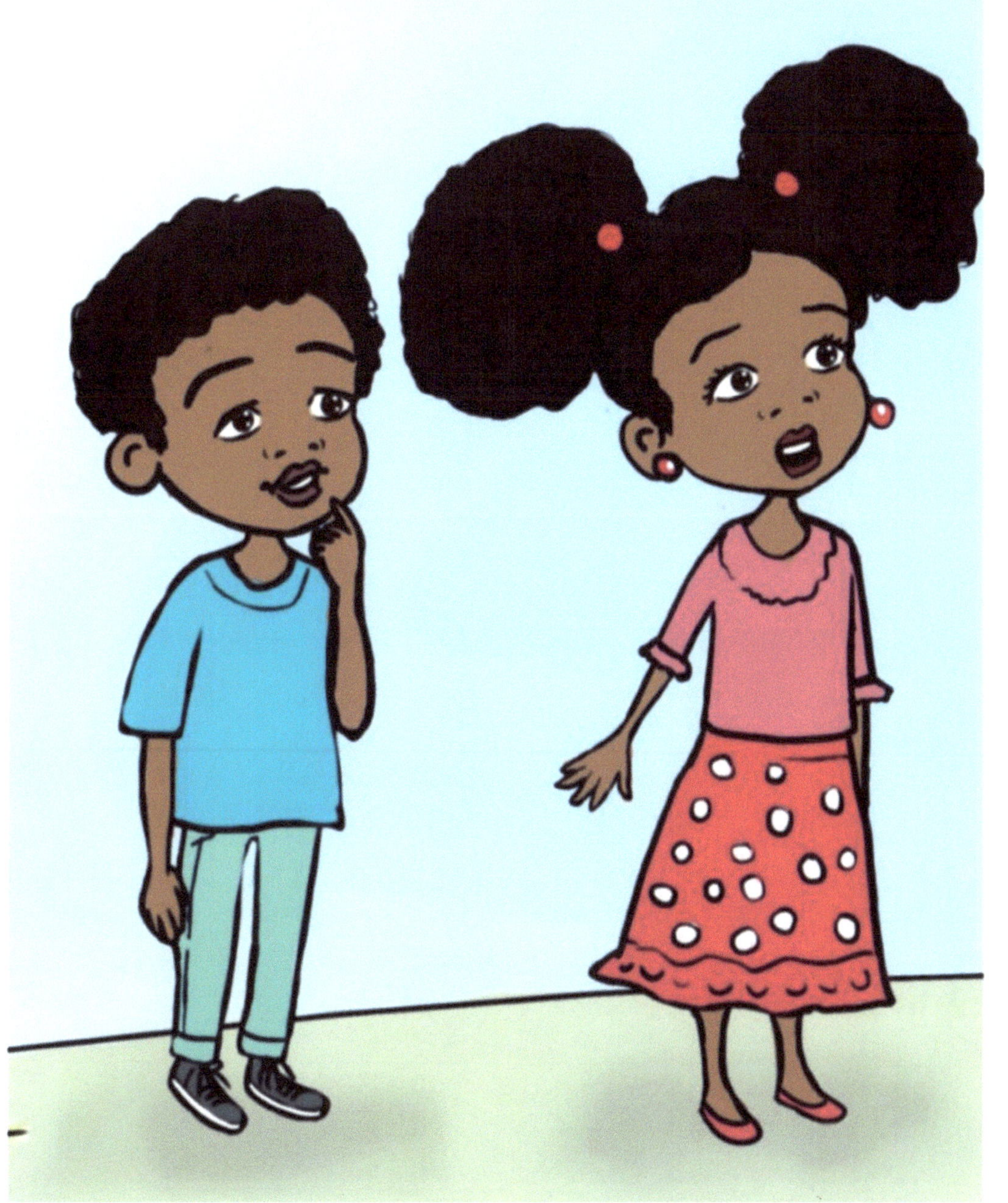

I am going to lay down in a few minutes, but first I need to help pack your bags for your grandparent's house.

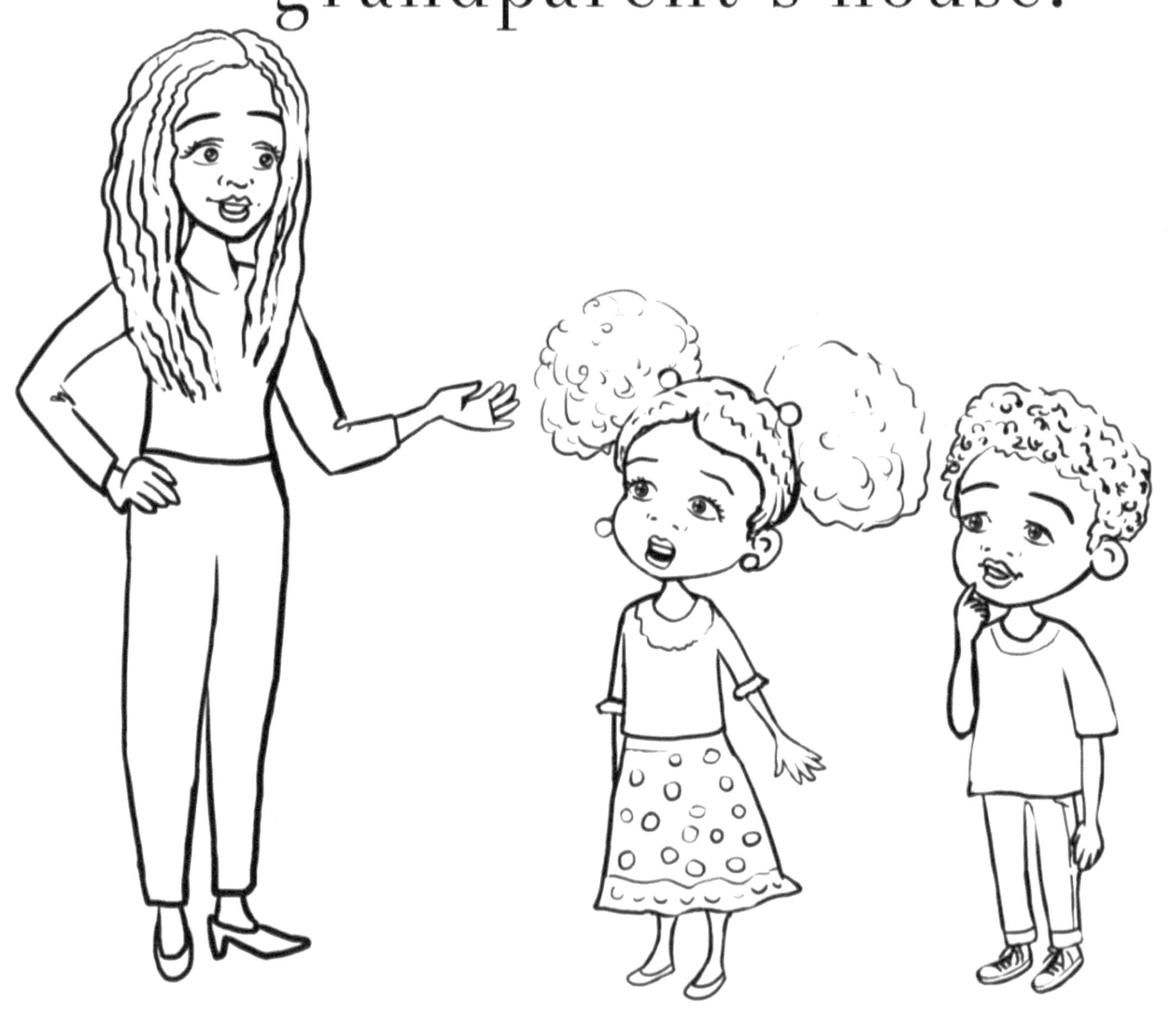

GRANDMA AND GRANDPA
HOUSE

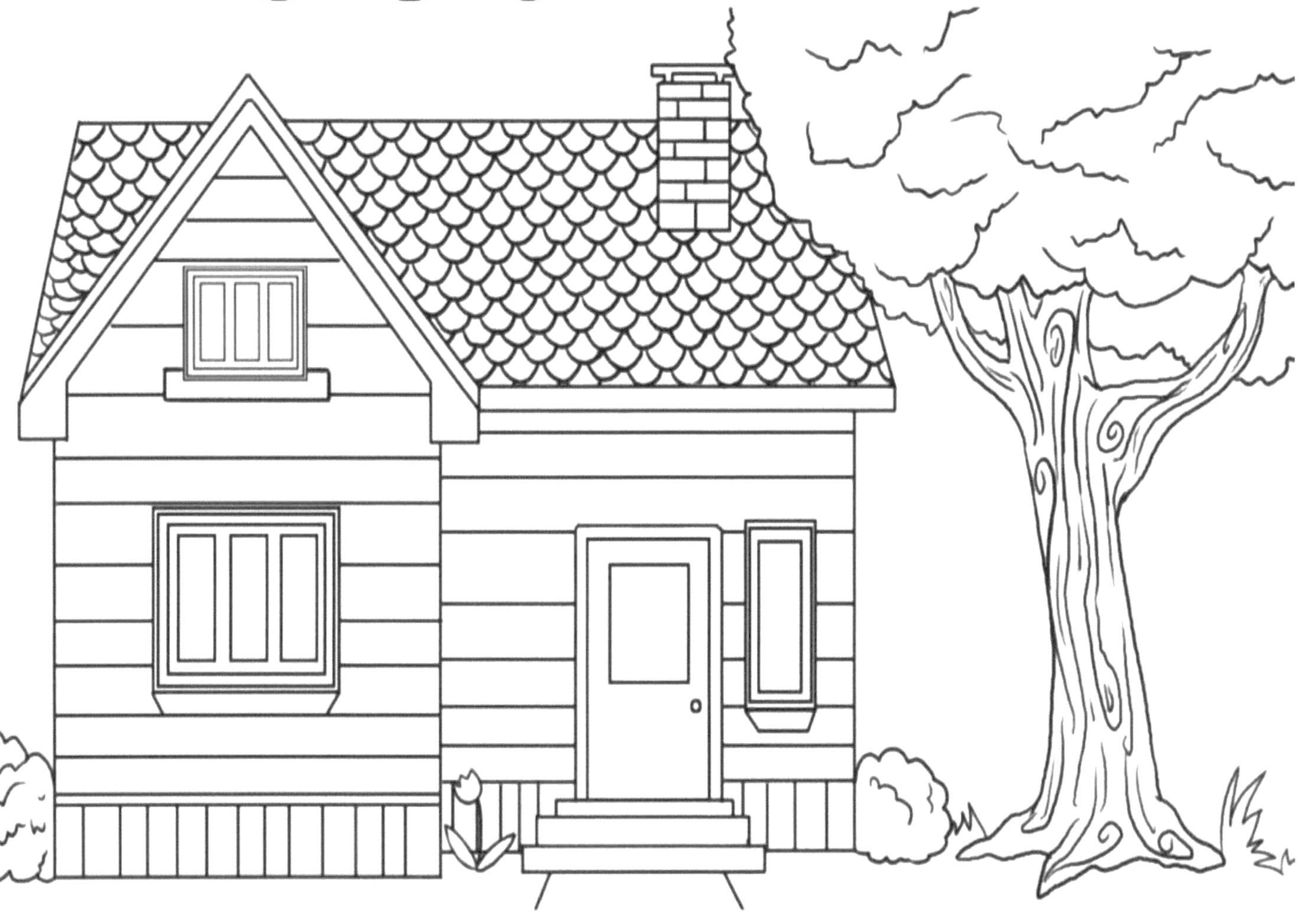

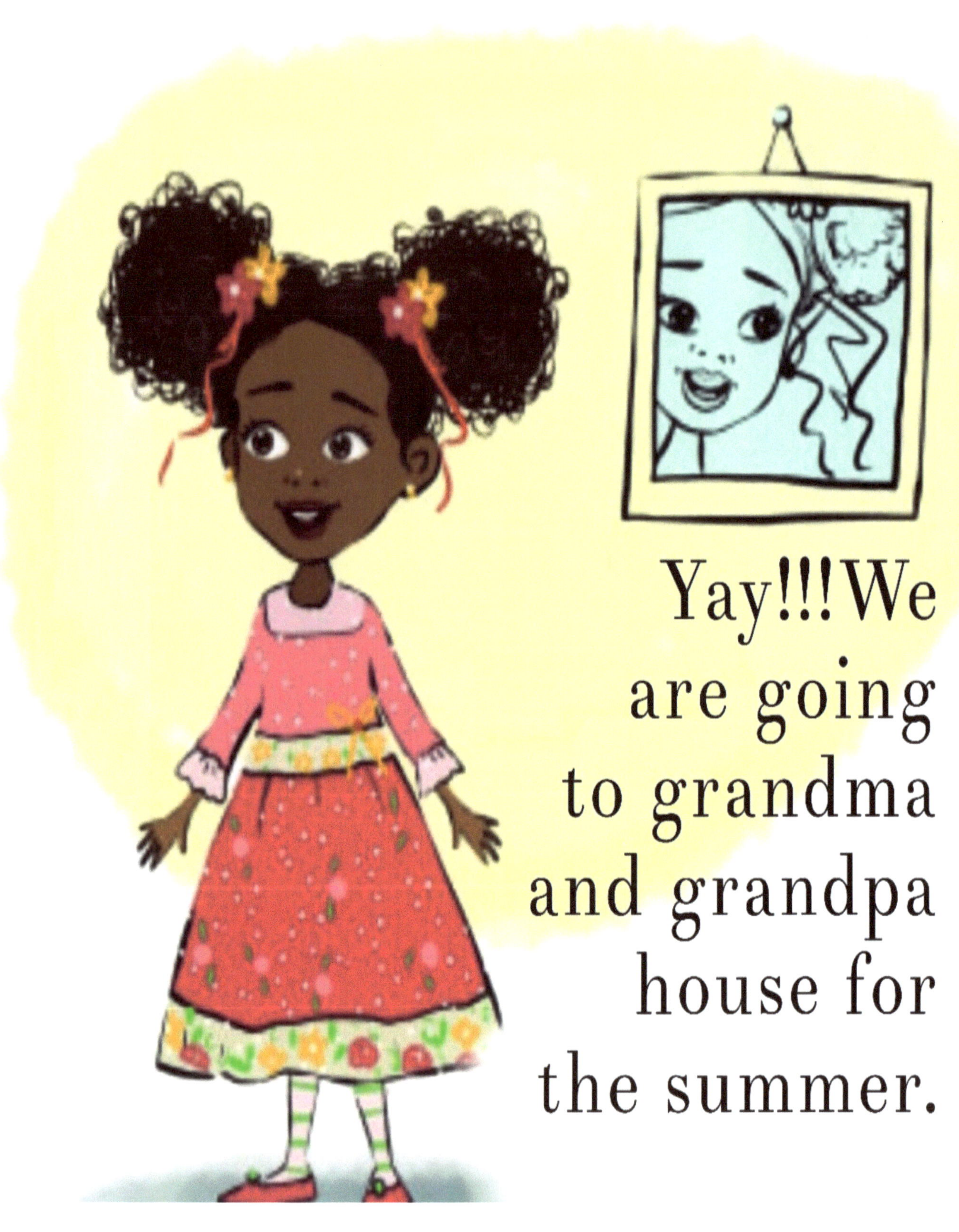

Yay!!!We
are going
to grandma
and grandpa
house for
the summer.

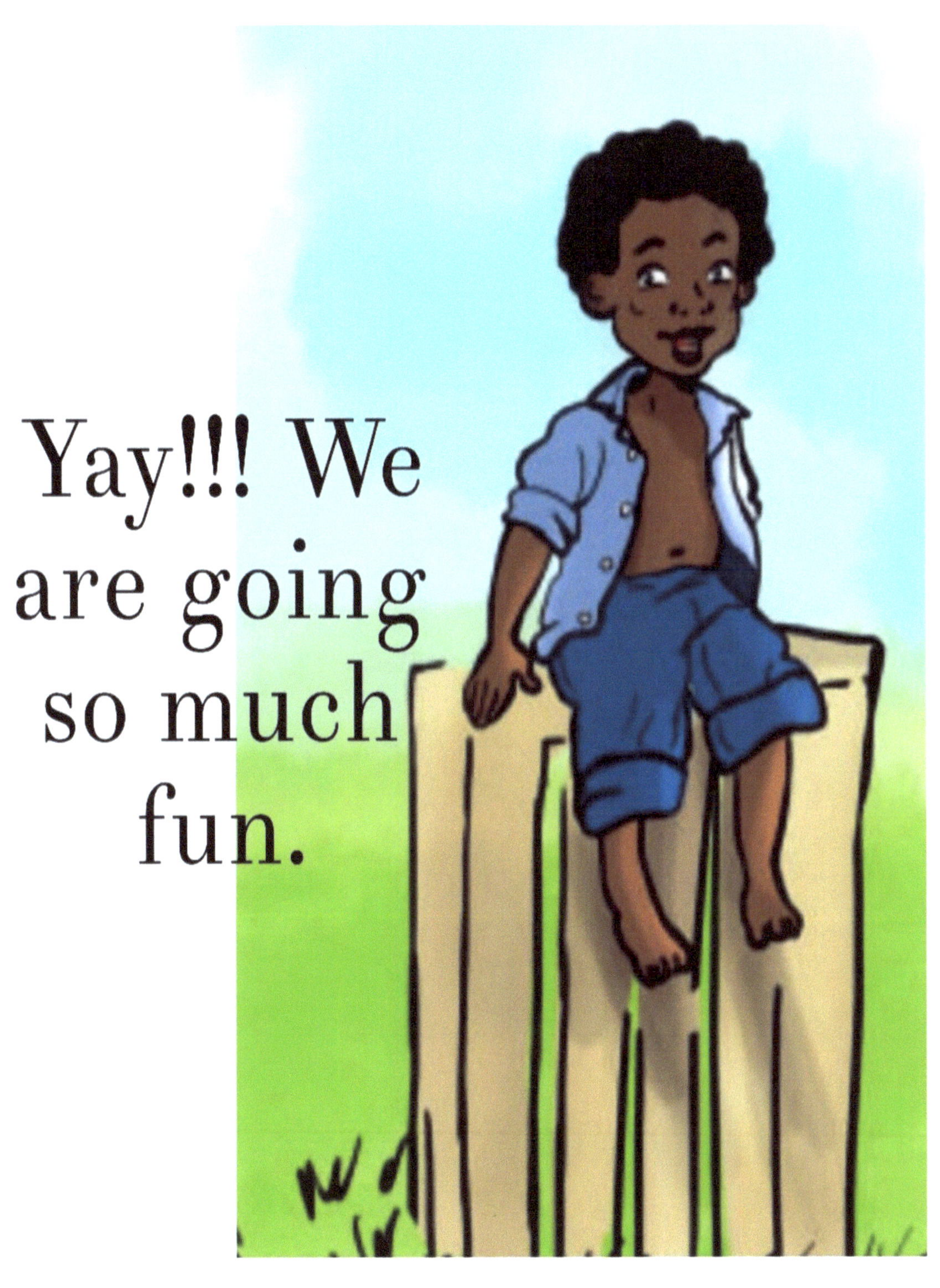

Yay!!! We are going so much fun.

Sara and Carter travelled to their grandparents for the summer while their mother, Wendy, deals with Breast Cancer. They road in their grandparents car.

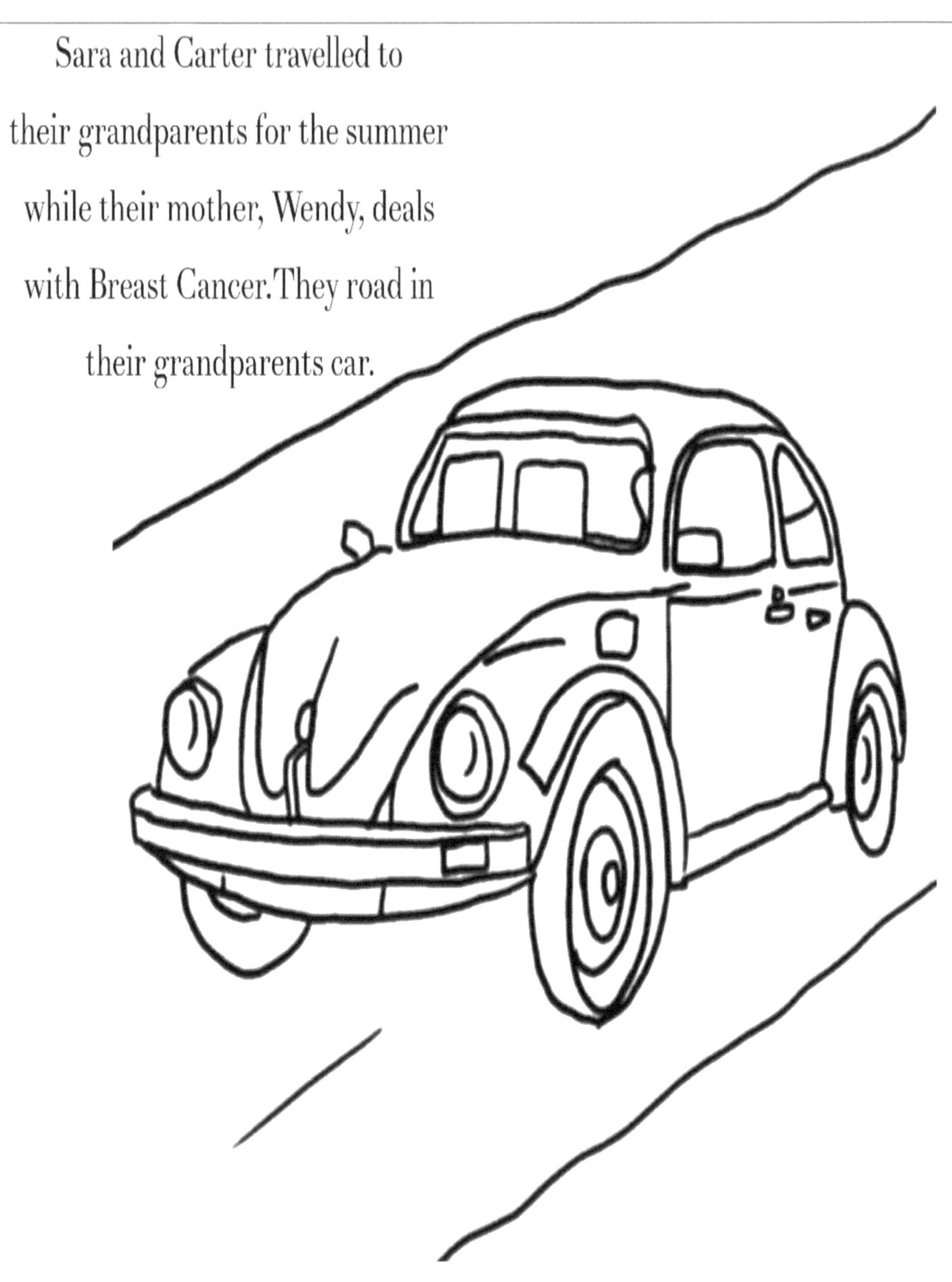

Wendy, Sara and
Carter mom, goes
to the doctor
in order to get
better.Her doctor
name is Dr. Kirol.

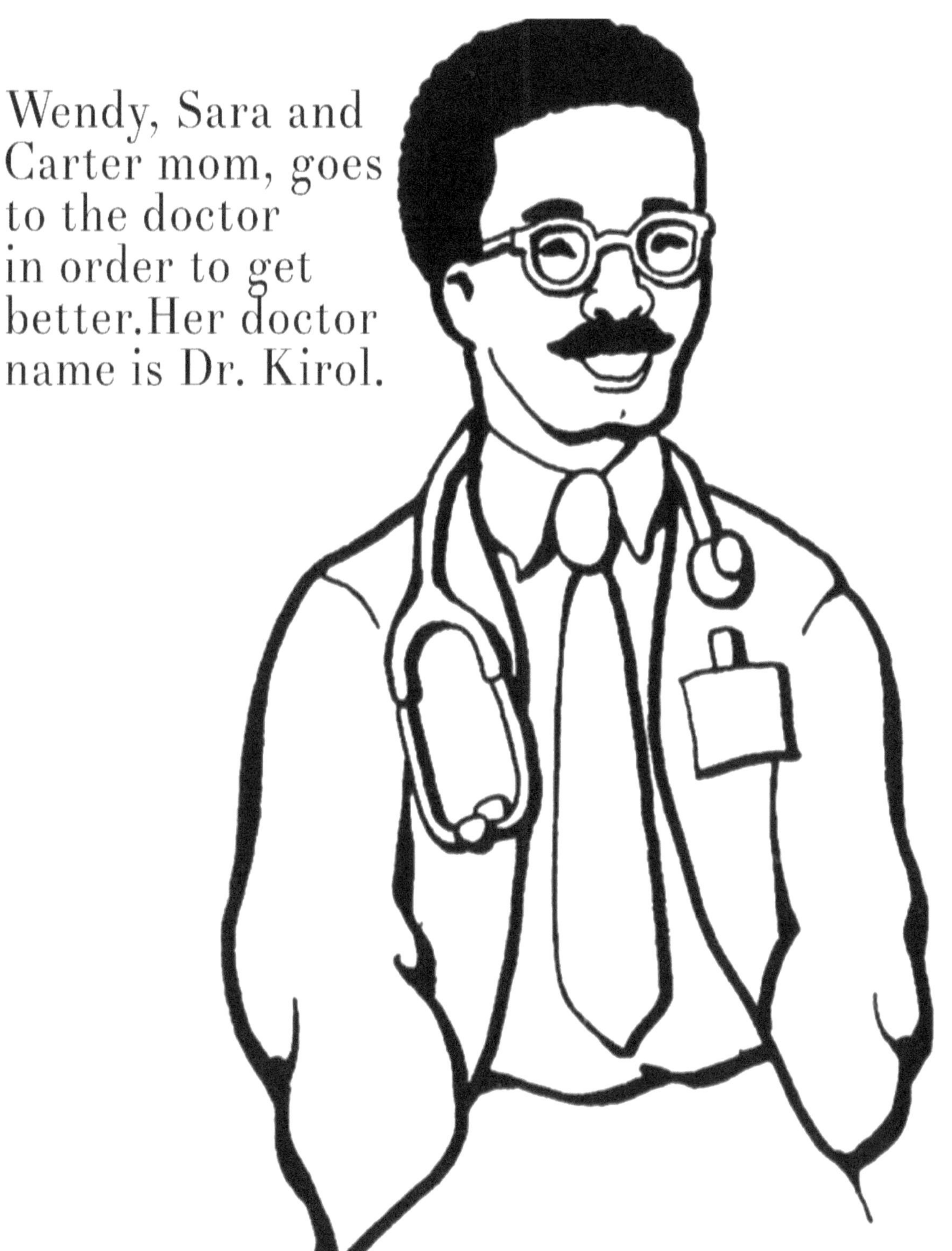

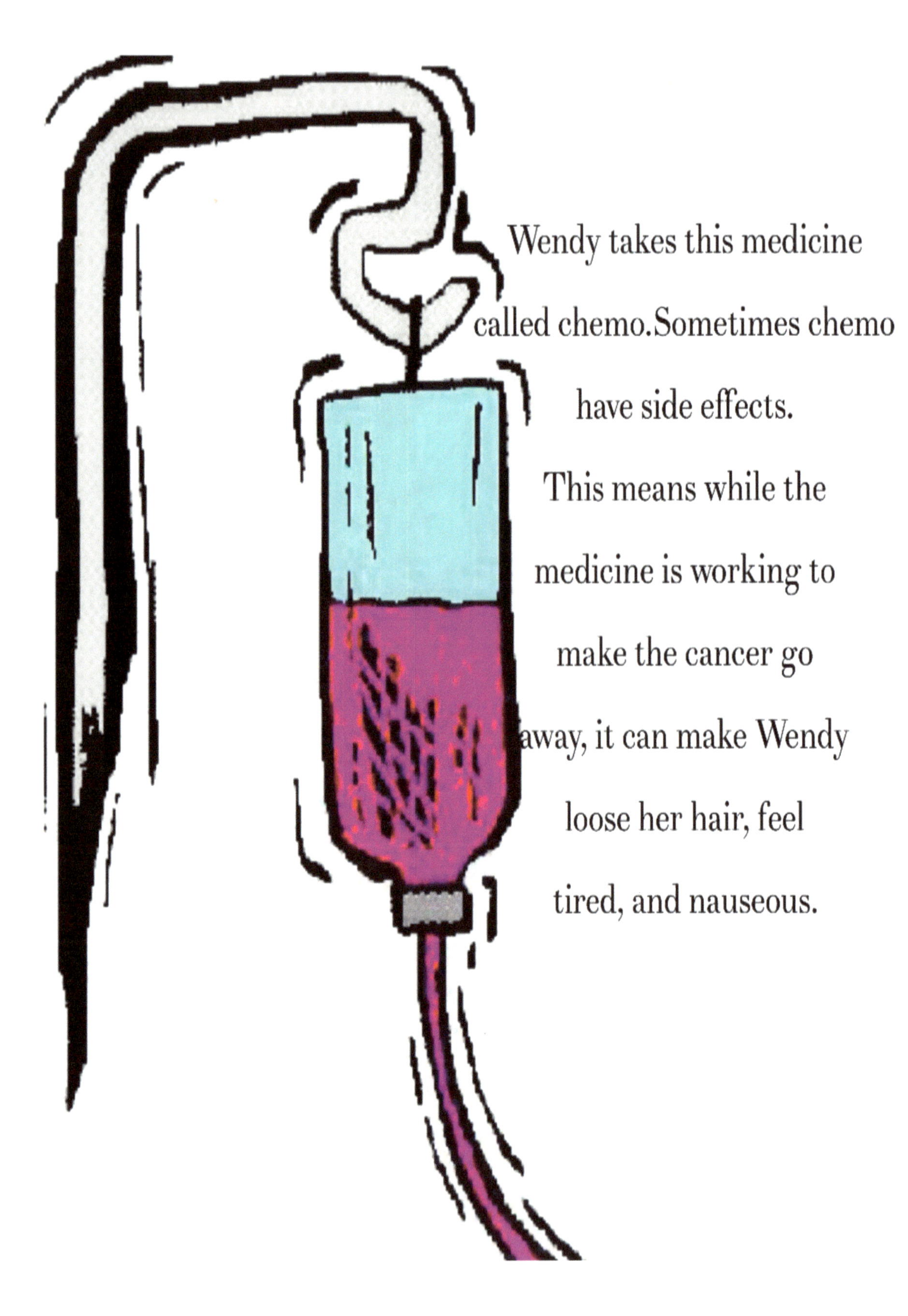

Wendy takes this medicine called chemo.Sometimes chemo have side effects. This means while the medicine is working to make the cancer go away, it can make Wendy loose her hair, feel tired, and nauseous.

The battle begin when
Wendy found the breast
cancer within. So,
Wendy started taking
the medicine.
Summer was coming to
a near end.Wendy had
begun having the side
effects to the medication.
She lost her long
dreadlocks.She was
sad.However, she knew her
hair would grow back with time.

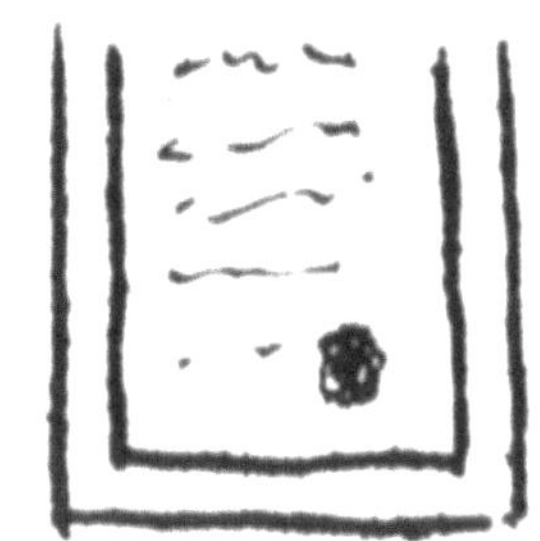

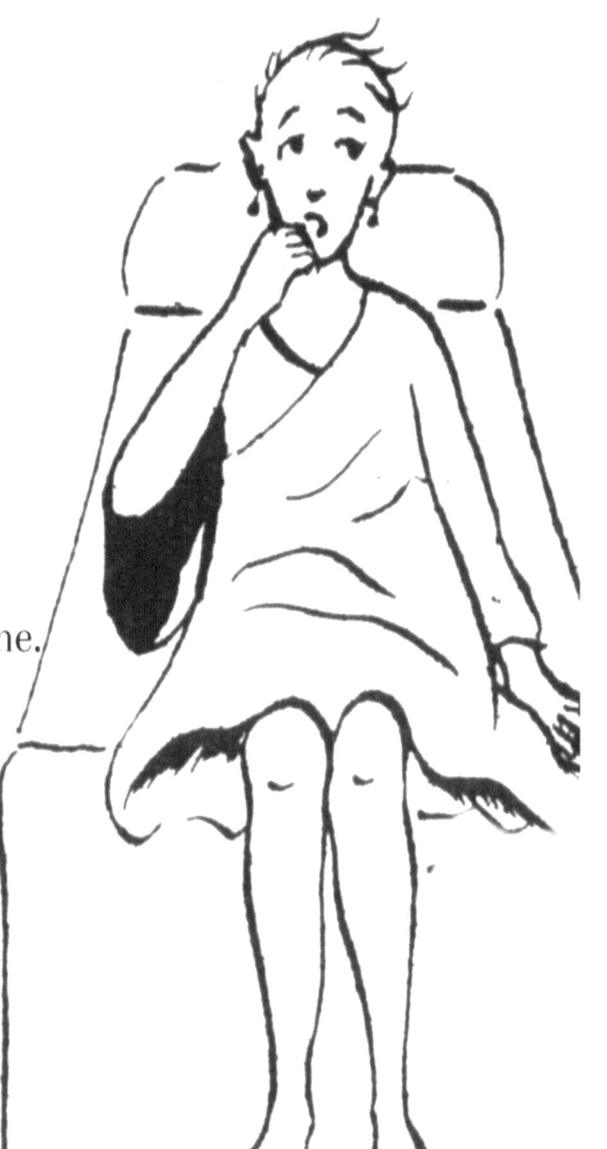

FOUR WIGS

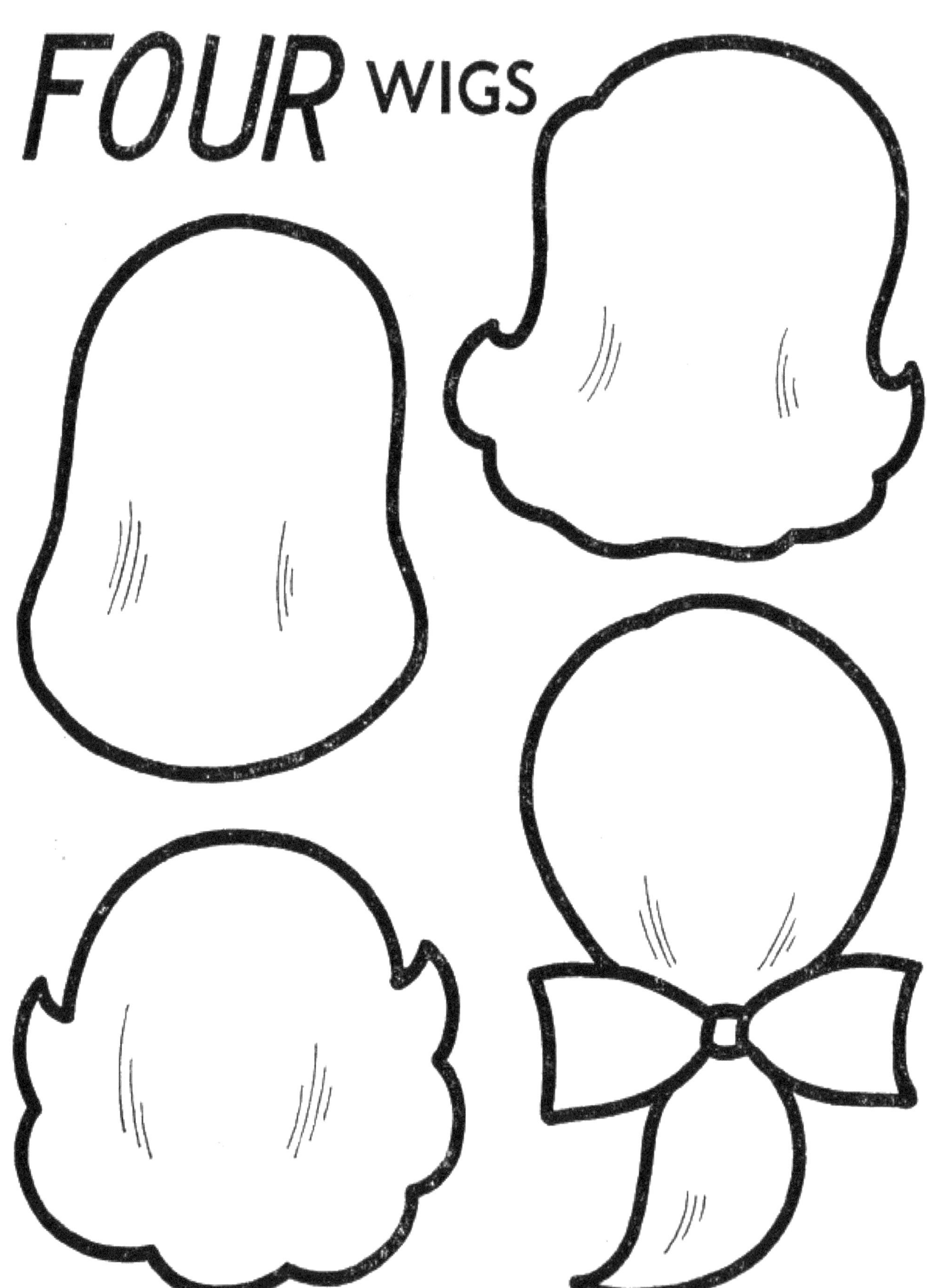

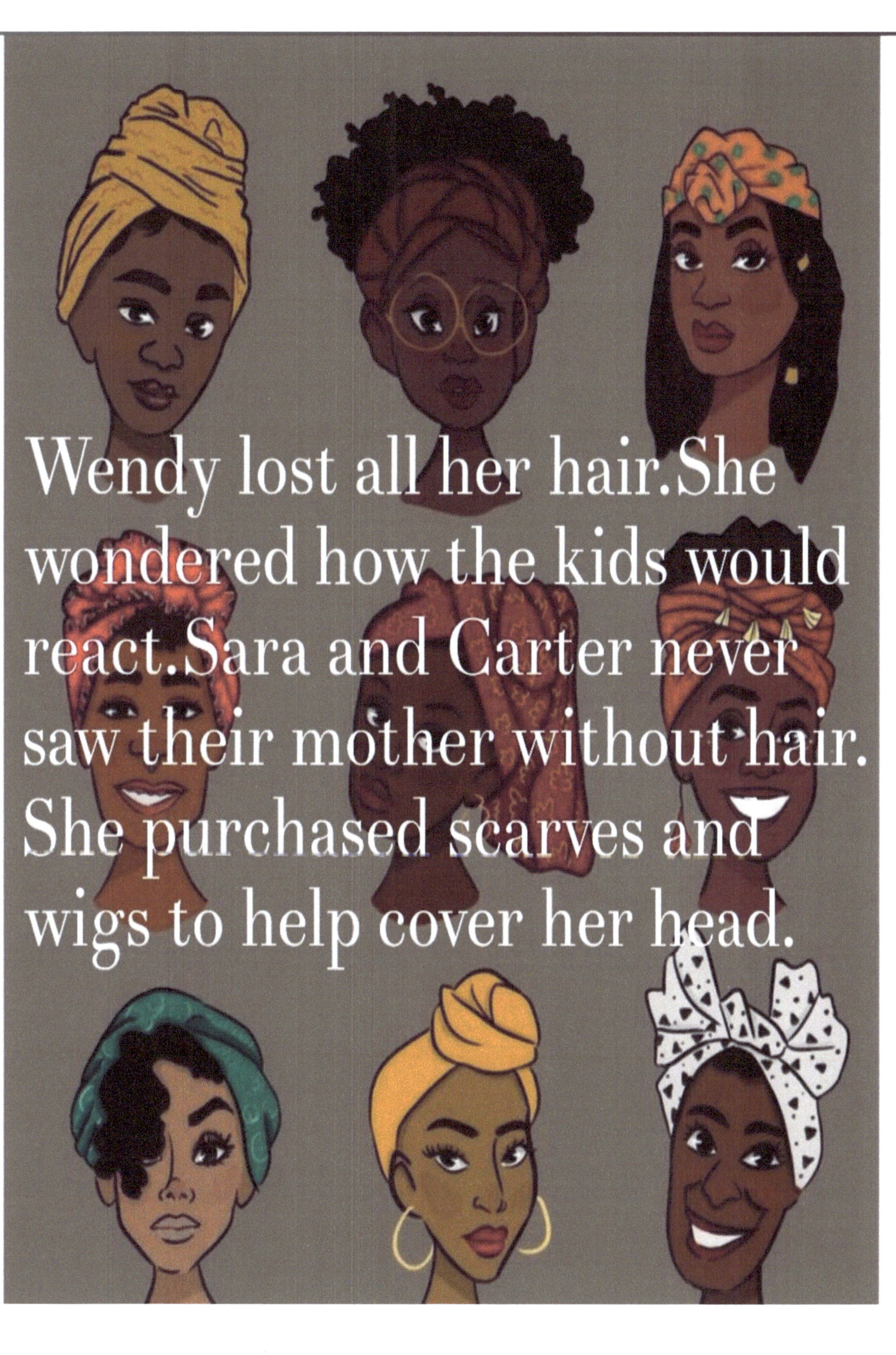

Wendy lost all her hair.She wondered how the kids would react.Sara and Carter never saw their mother without hair. She purchased scarves and wigs to help cover her head.

Wendy was scheduled to have the cancer removed. That meant she had to have her boob removed. Not only did she lost her hair, but she lost her boob. She was nervous about seeing the kids in a few weeks. She had heard that they had so much fun with her parents.

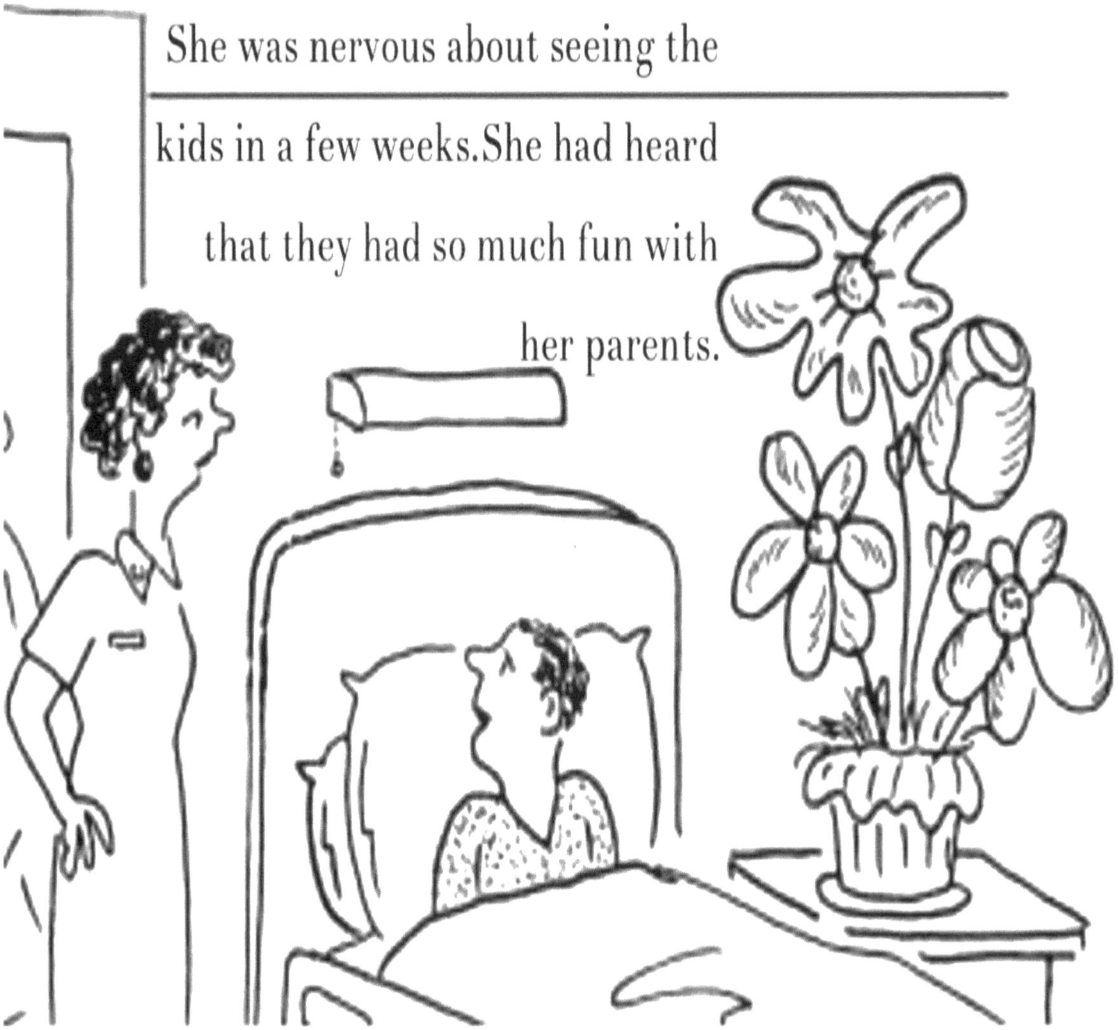

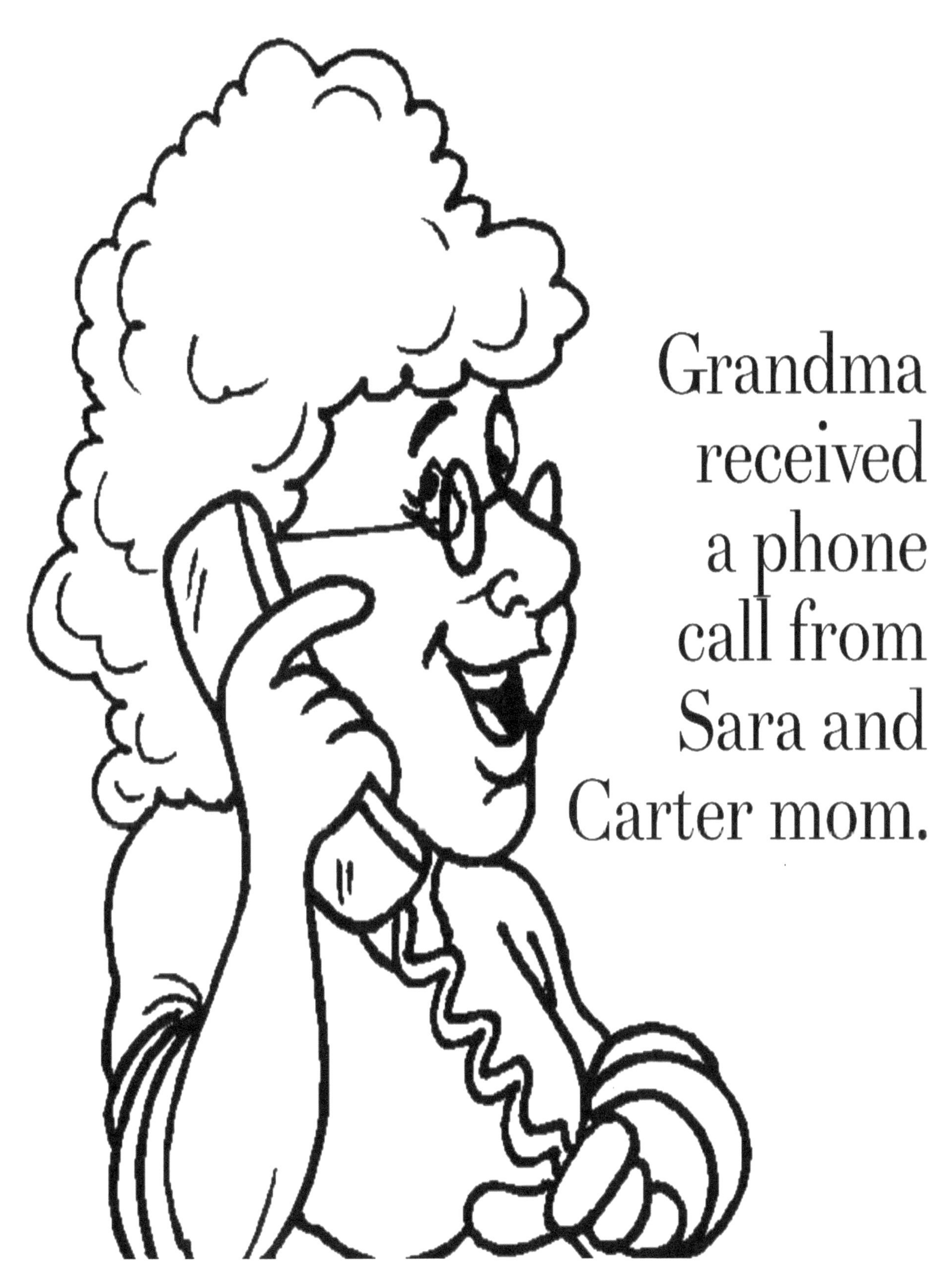

Grandma
received
a phone
call from
Sara and
Carter mom.

Wendy told Sara and Carter grandma
on the phone to get them both prepared
to come home.Sara and Carter were
excited to get back home to their mommy.

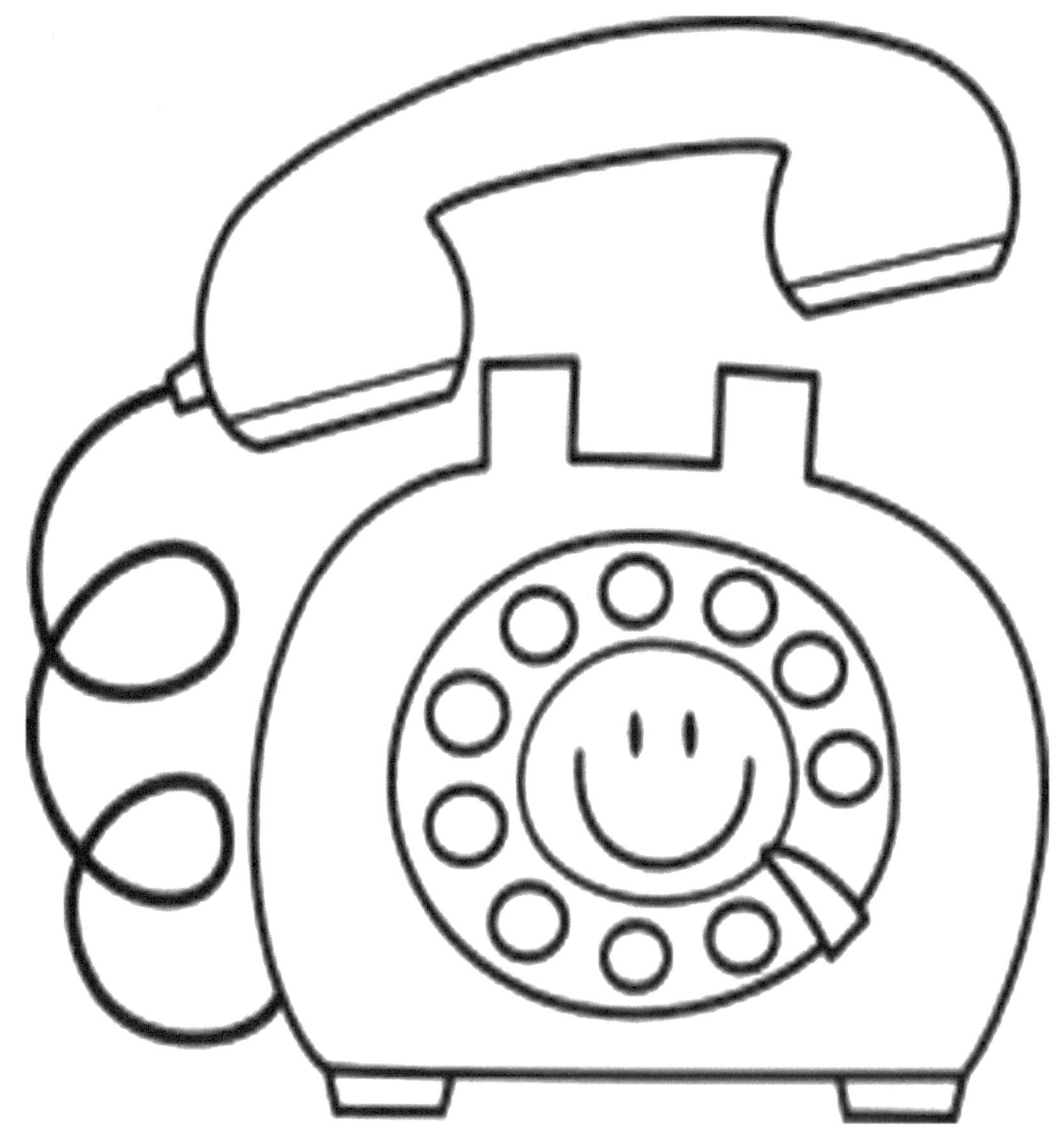

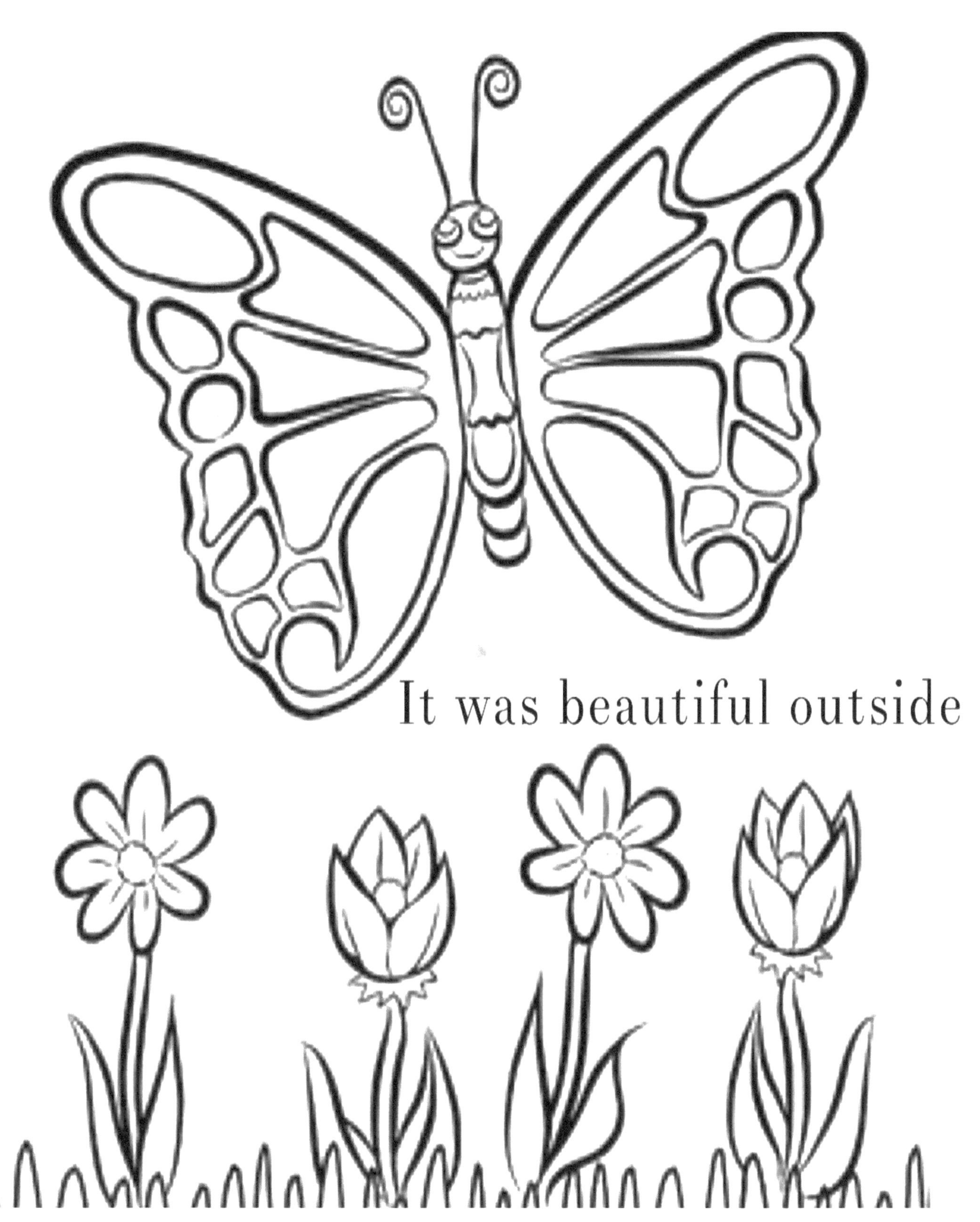

It was beautiful outside

Sara and Carter arrives back

home.They both stood outside yelling

mommy mommy mommy.

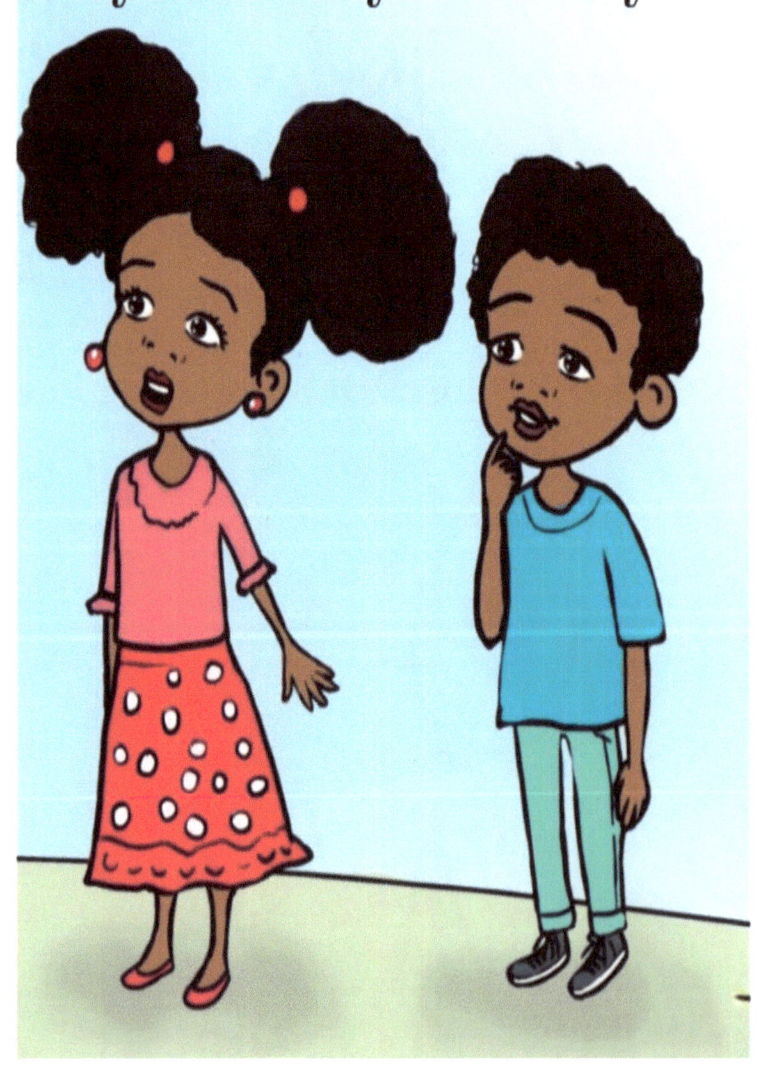

Sara
and
Carter
had
gifts
to give
to their mom.

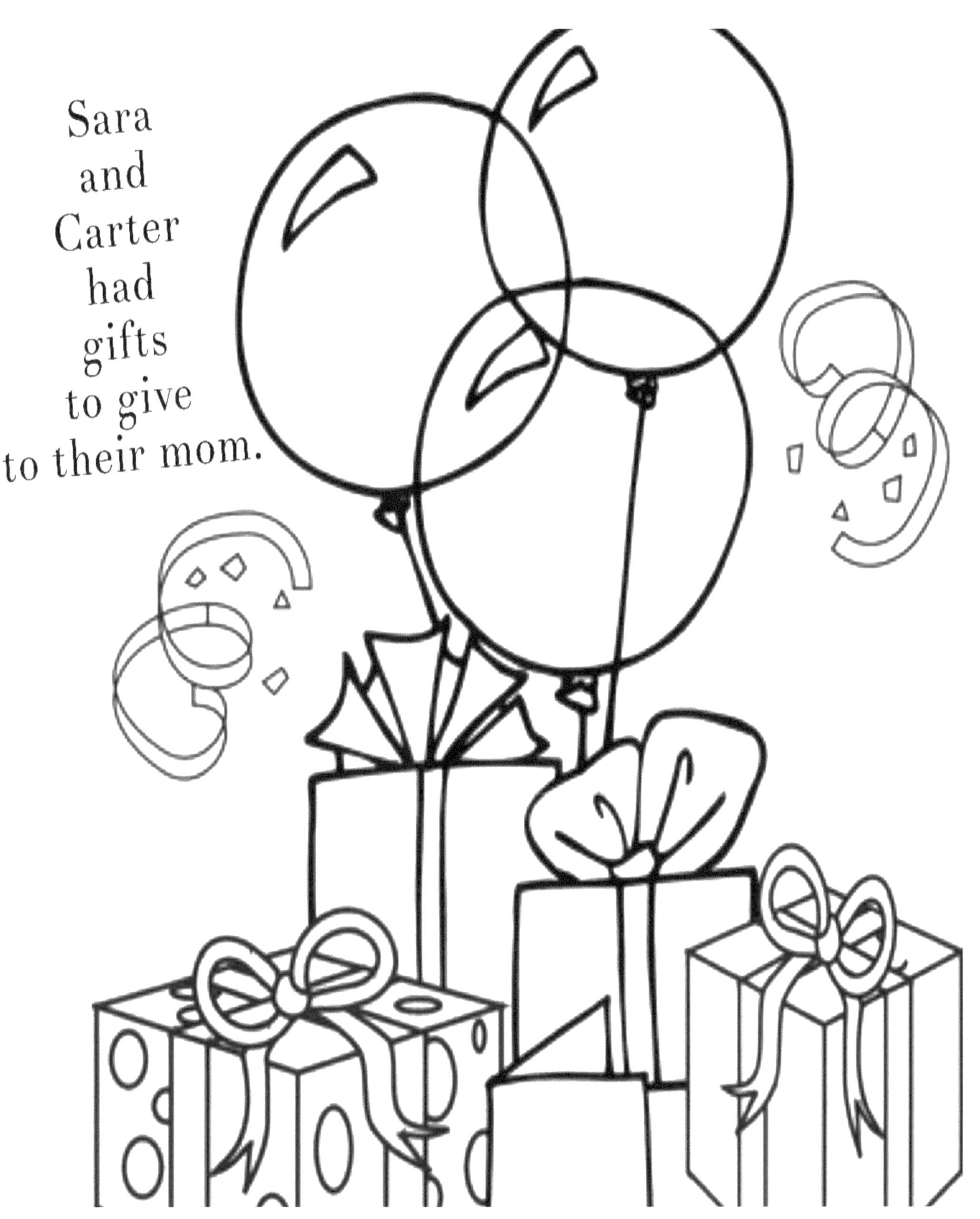

Wendy heard Sara and Carter because the front door was open.She yelled I am in my room kids come in the house

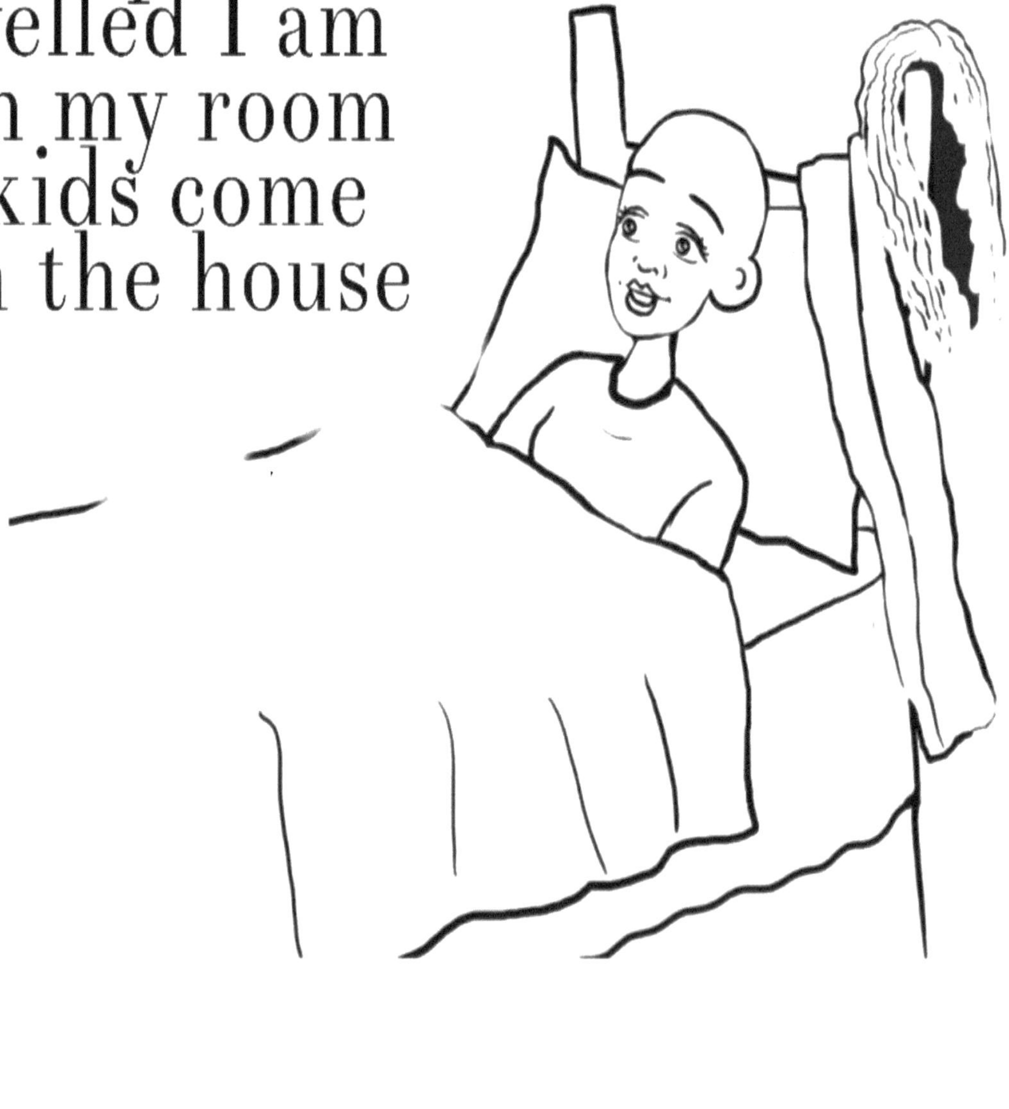

They saw their mom lying in bed.
Carter asked "Mommy what is
wrong?Do you feel okay?What
happened to your hair?"

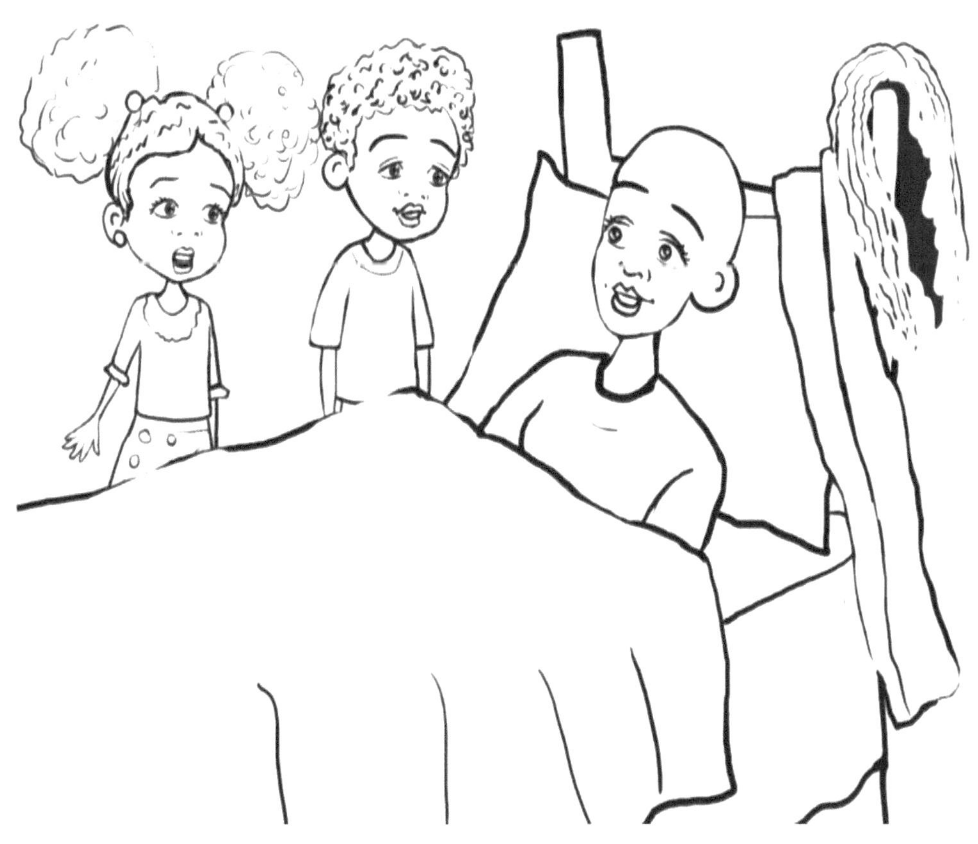

She replied, I am a little tired. The medicine I had to take to help the boo boo in my boob caused me to lose my hair and my boob.
That's breast cancer for you!

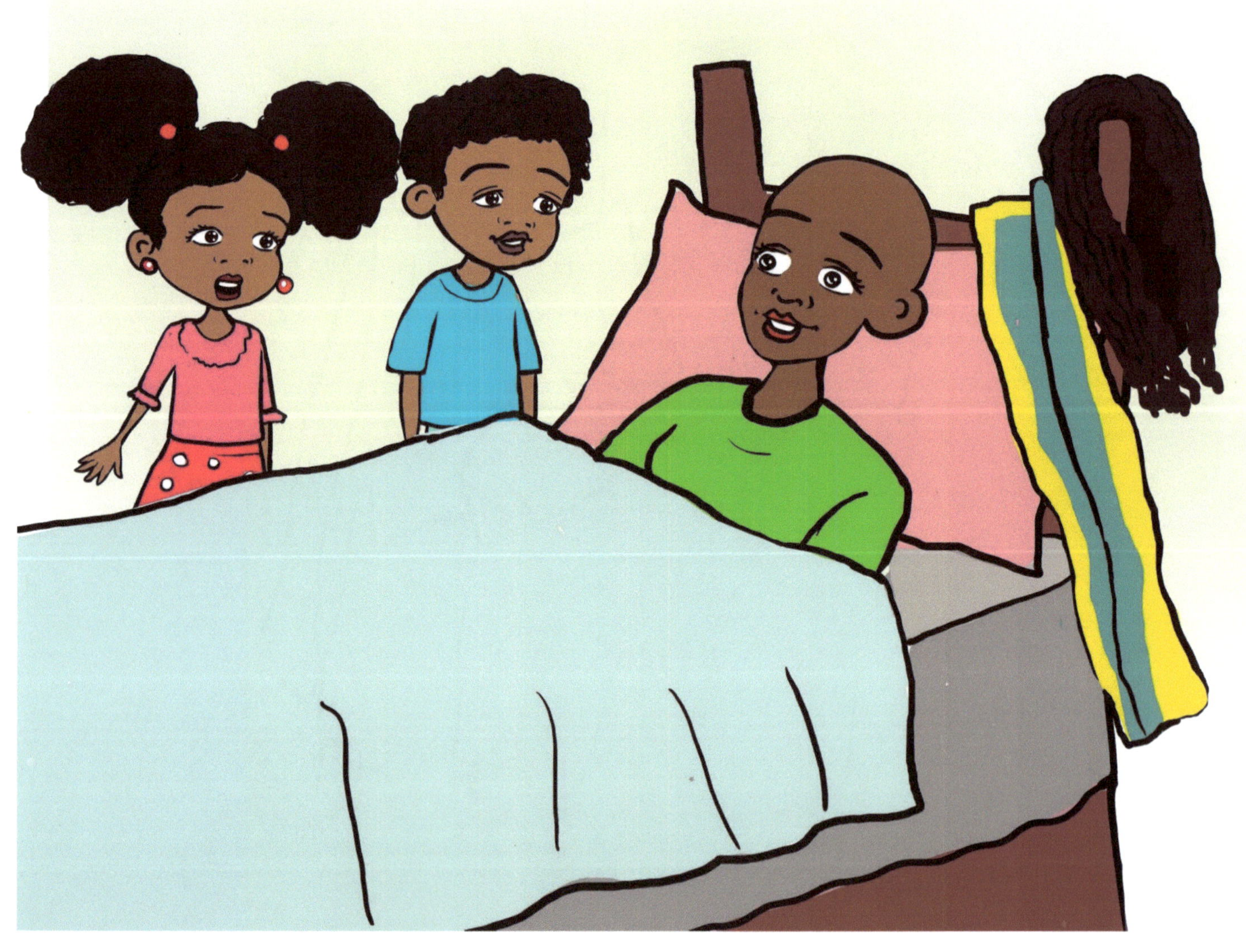

Mom, we hope that you feel better.

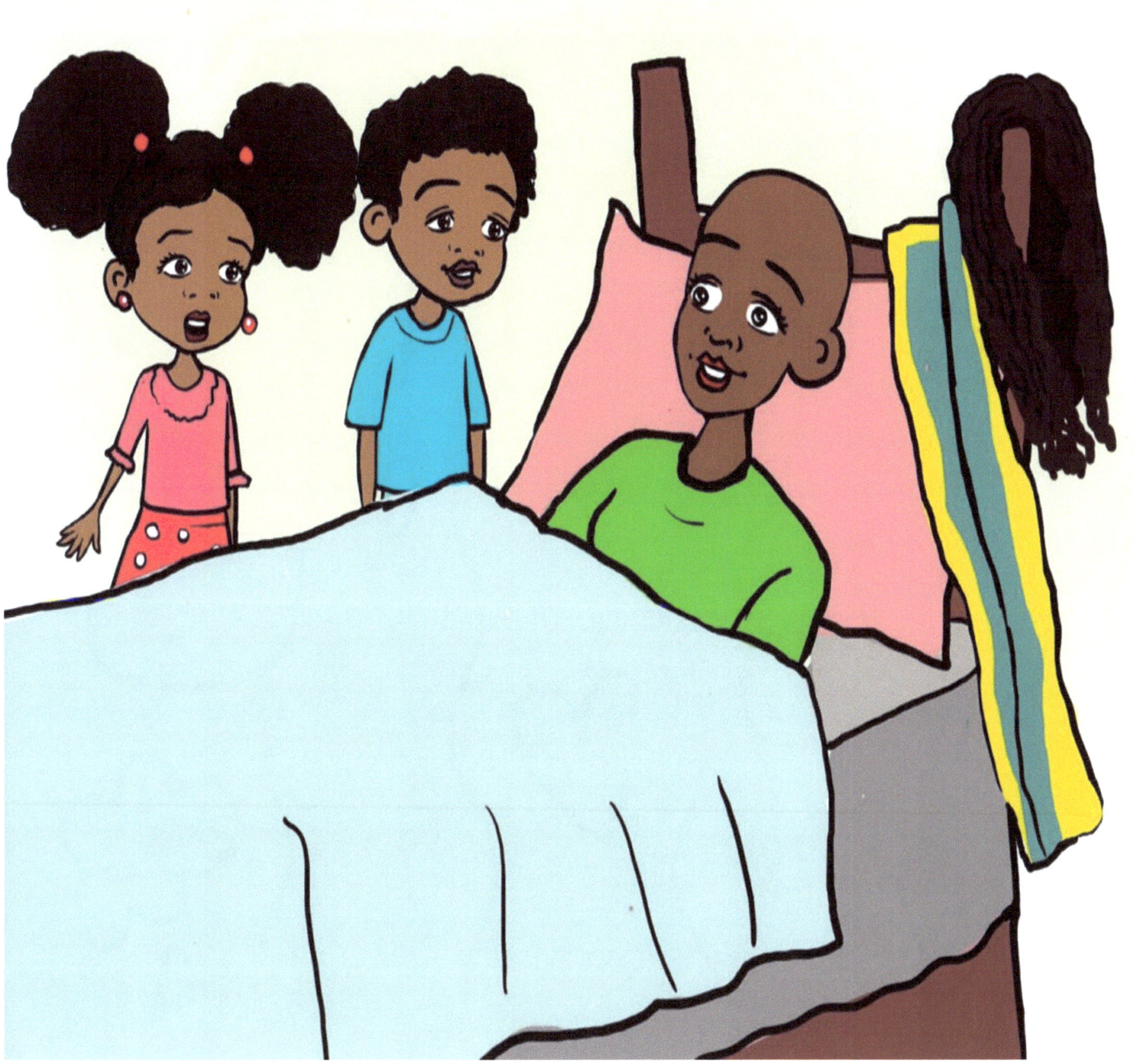

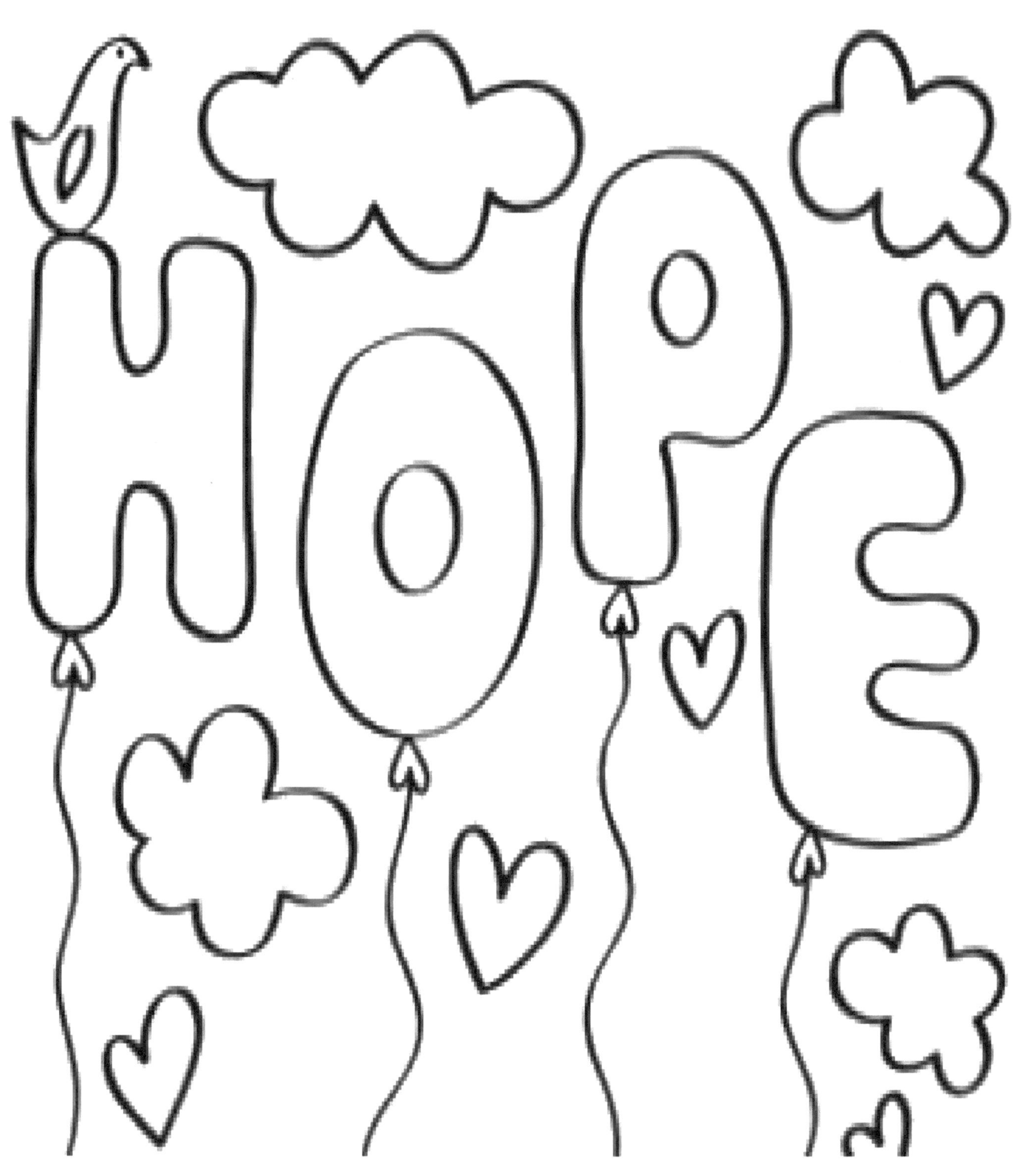

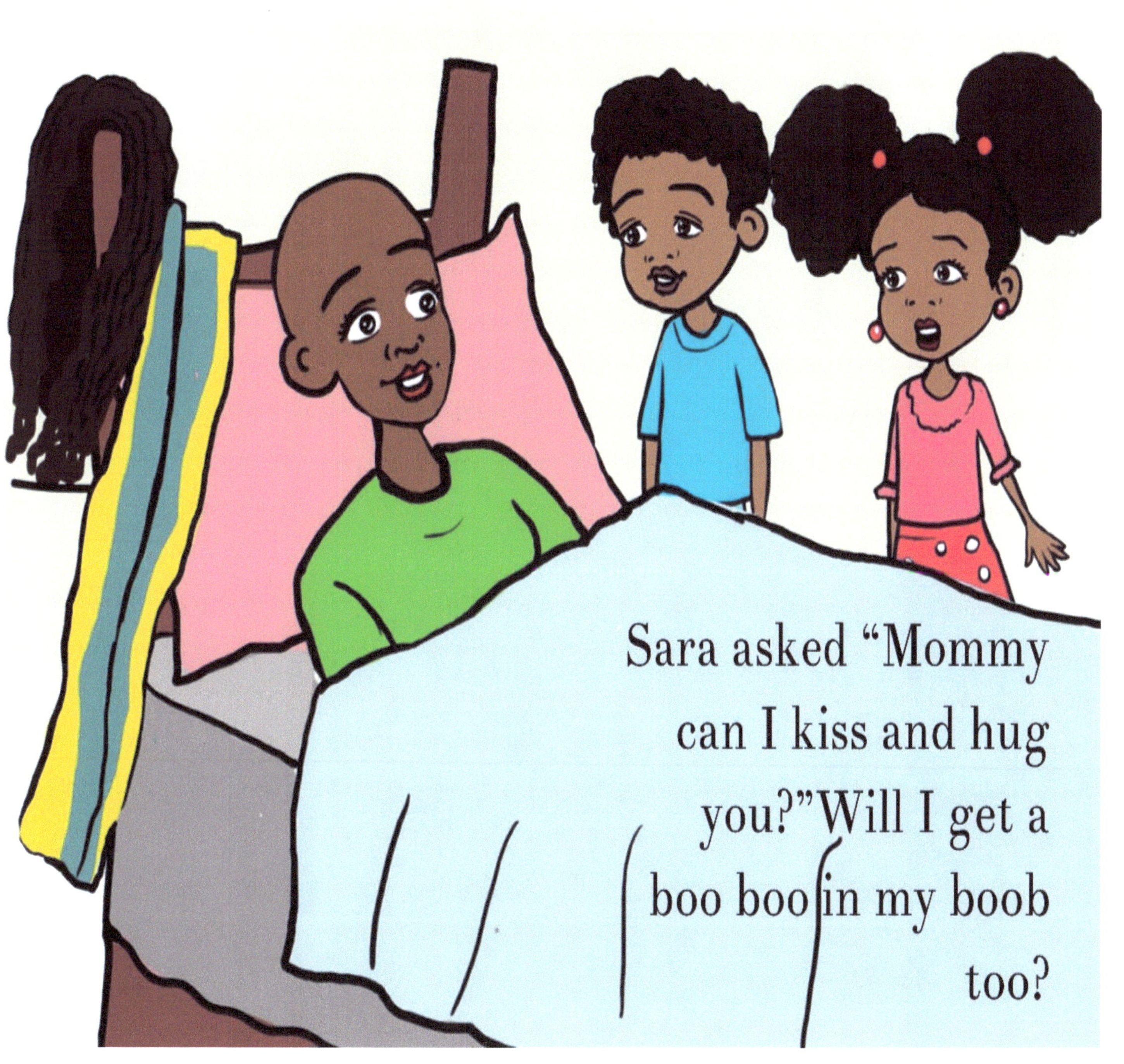

Sara asked "Mommy can I kiss and hug you?"Will I get a boo boo in my boob too?

No Sara you cannot catch breast
cancer from hugging and kissing
mommy. Besides you don't even
have a boob.So you can still
hug and kiss mommy.In fact,
kissing and hugging me will make
me happy.

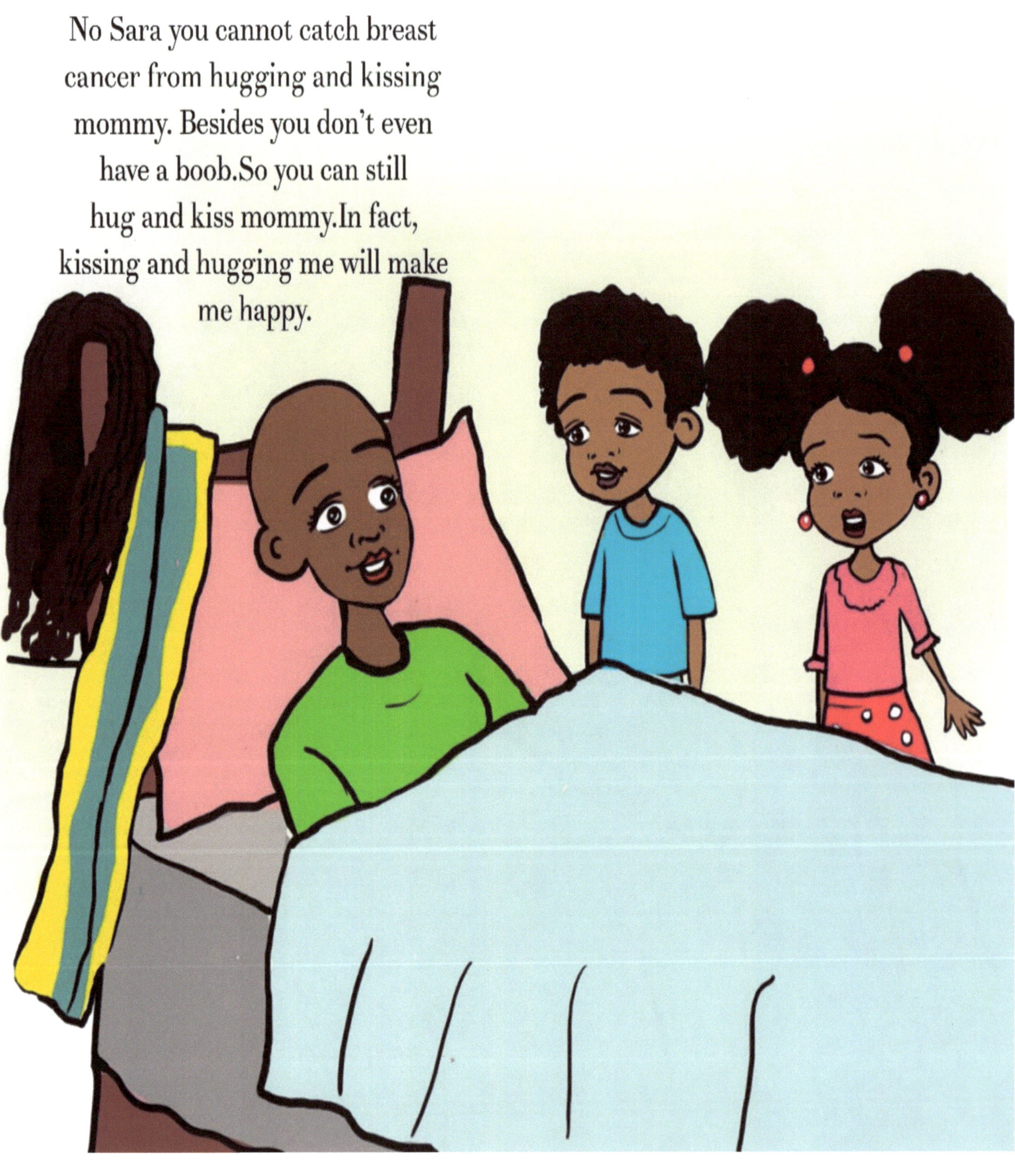

Mommy lost her hair but my
smile is still there.I had to
say goodbye to my boob so I
could be here with you.Now I
feel better.
Cancer came took my hair and
my boob, but it did not take
me away from you.It was hard
but I fought back even harder
because I wanted to be here
with my Sara and Carter.

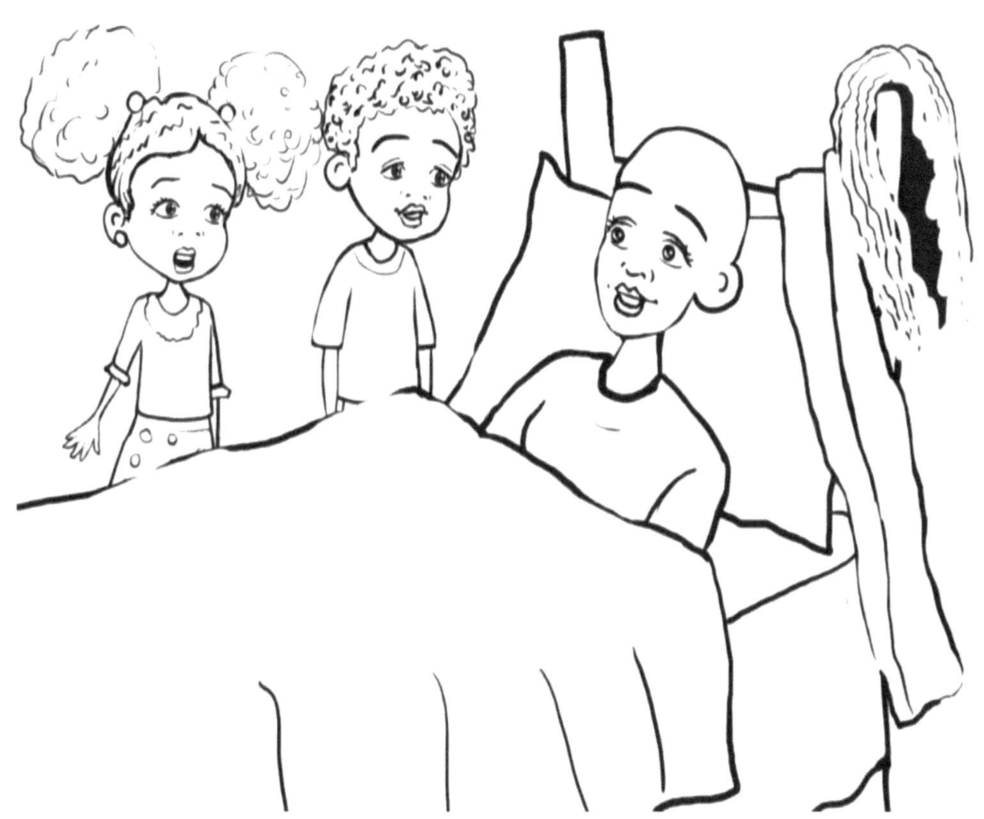

We are glad that you
are here with us too
mom. We love you mommy.

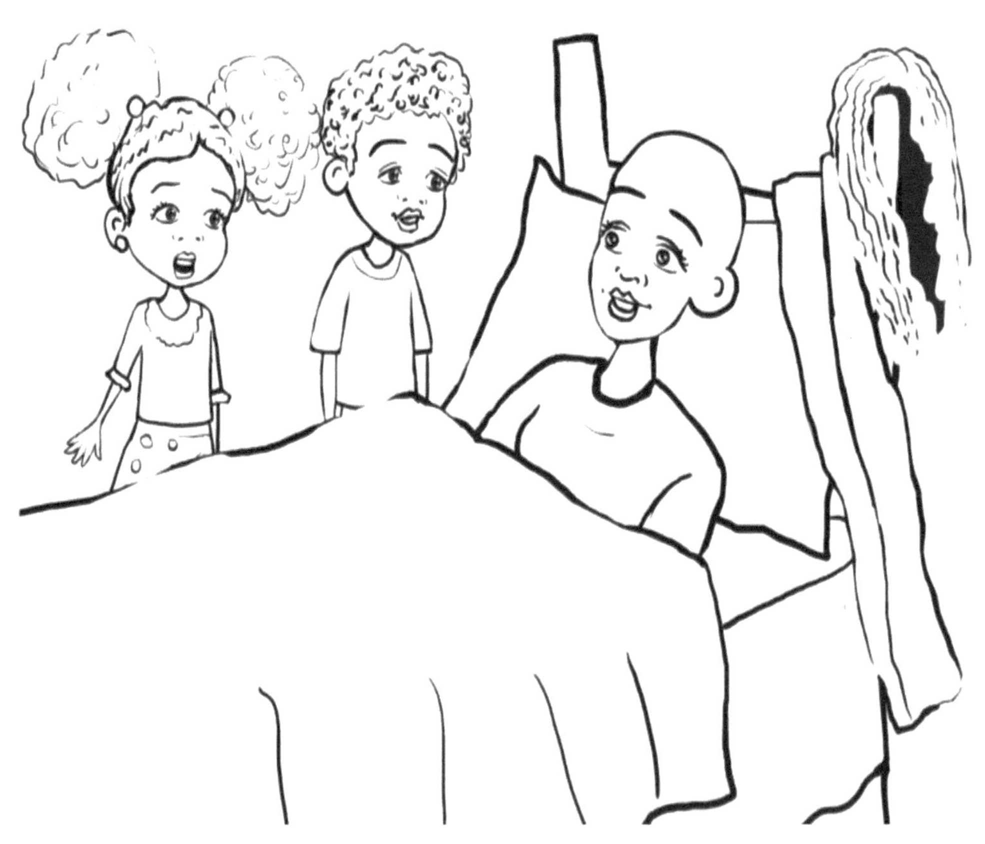

I love you too!God entrusted this
journey to me so that I can tell
the world How God healed me and
that He could do it for them.Cancer
took me by surprise, but not God.

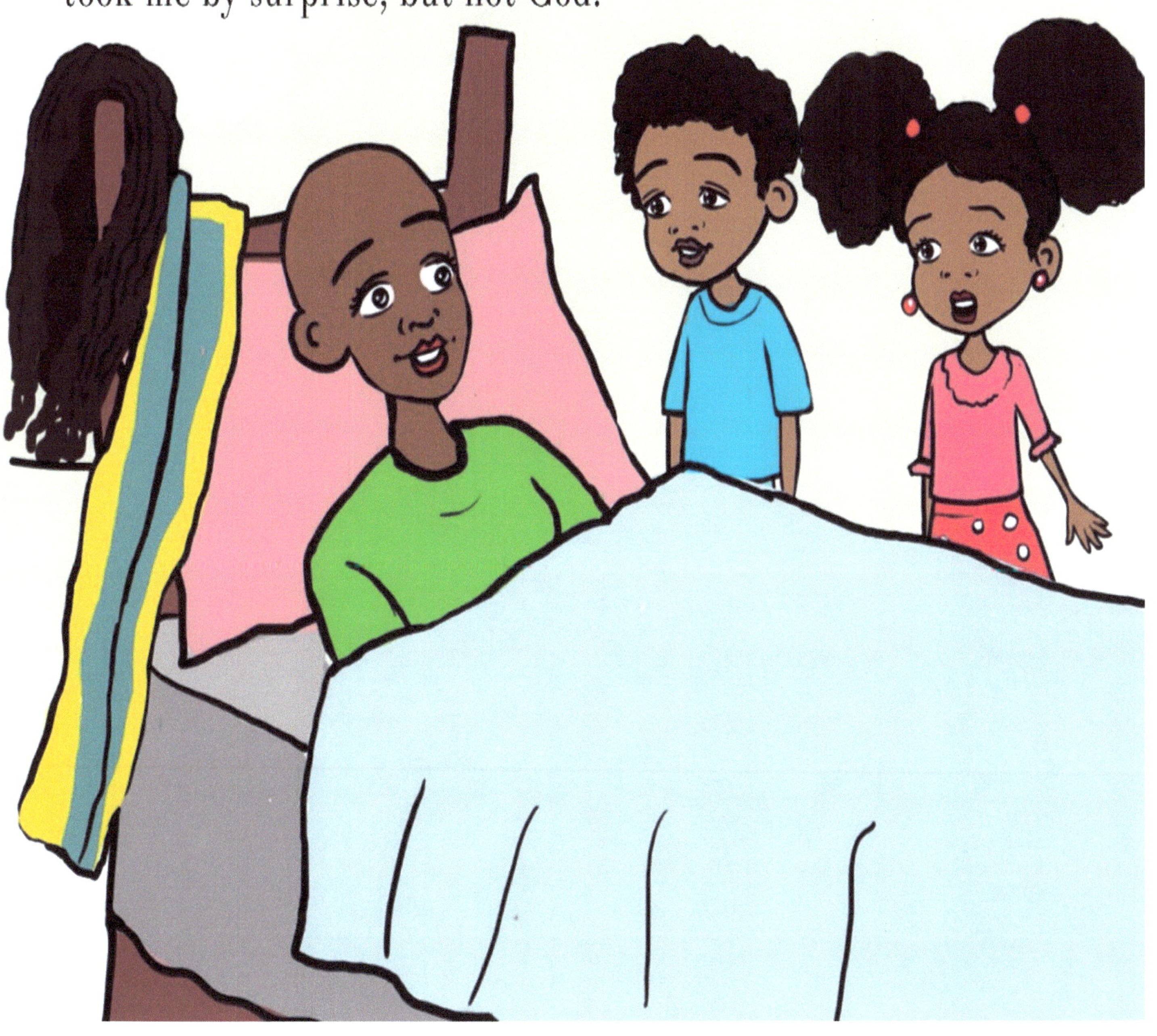

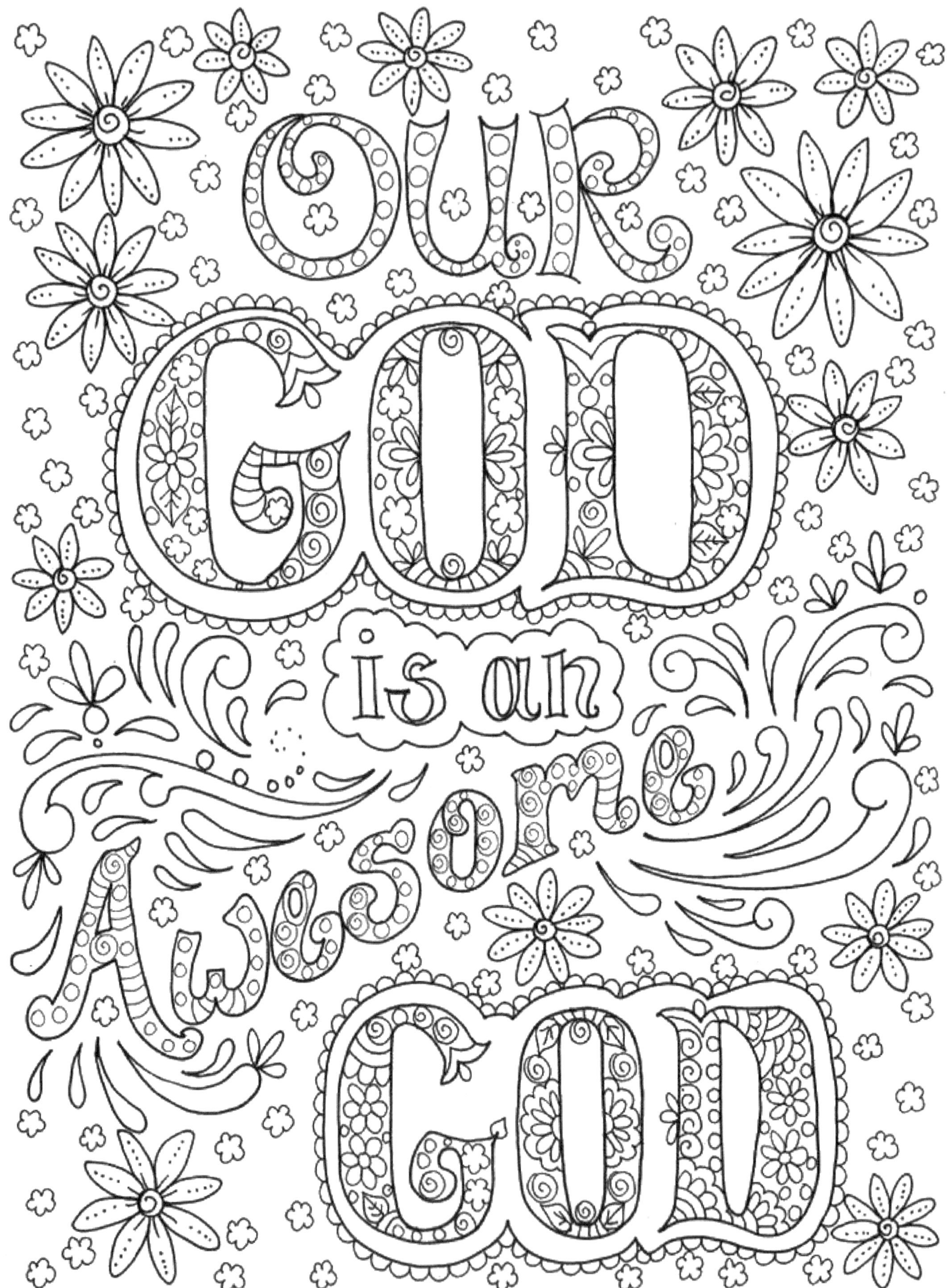

OUR
GOD
is an
Awesome
GOD

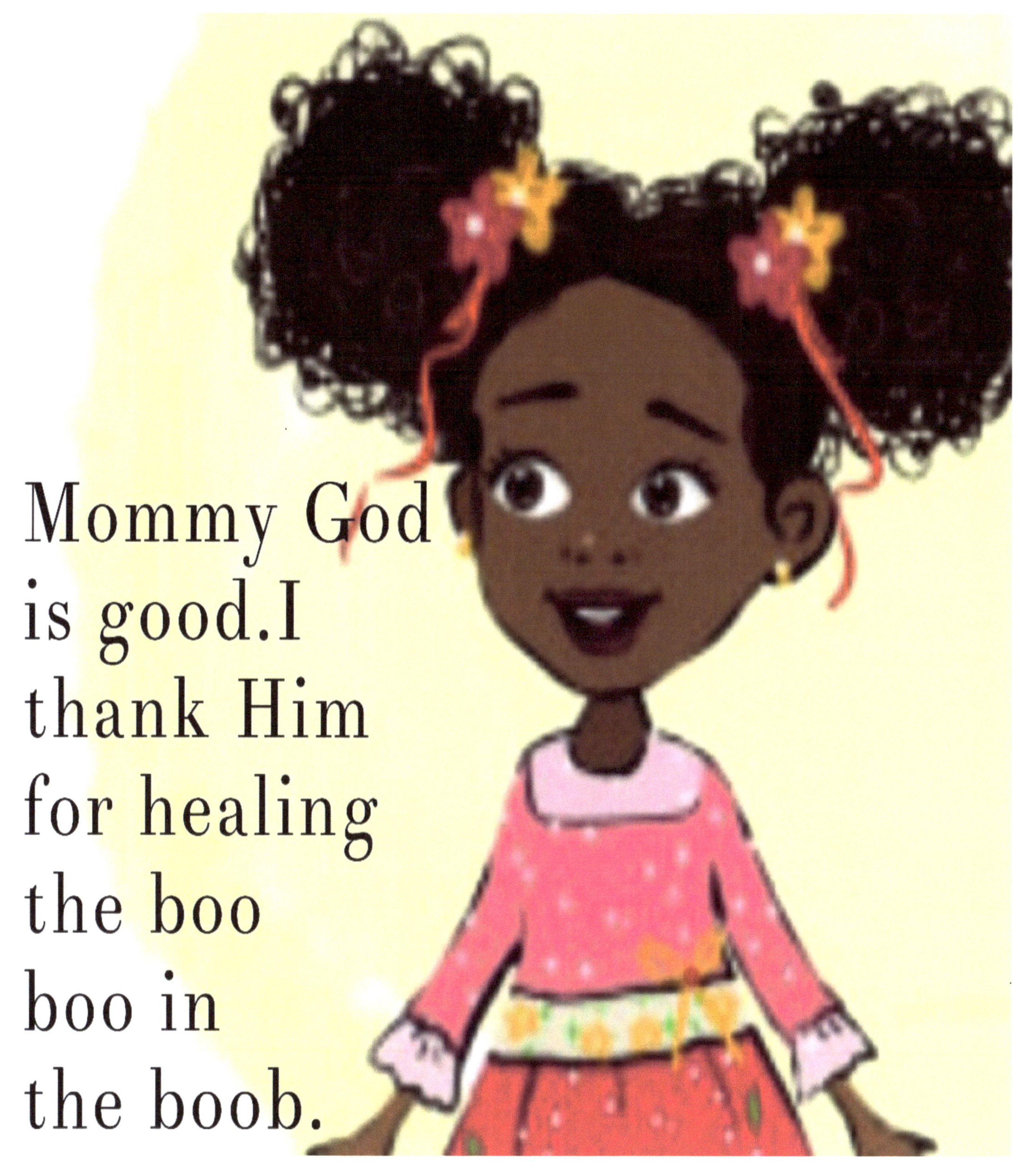

Mommy God is good. I thank Him for healing the boo boo in the boob.